Supplement to the Fifteenth Edition of
*Standard Methods for the Examination of
Water and Wastewater:*

SELECTED ANALYTICAL METHODS APPROVED AND CITED BY THE UNITED STATES ENVIRONMENTAL PROTECTION AGENCY

Prepared and Published by:

American Public Health Association
American Water Works Association
Water Pollution Control Federation

30M6/81
Library of Congress Catalog Number: 81-67882
International Standard Book Number: 0-87553-094-X

Printed and bound in the United States of America
  Text and Binding: Port City Press

090004

TABLE OF CONTENTS

METHODS

I. METALS

II. INORGANIC NON-METALS

III. ORGANIC COMPOUNDS
A. General
B. Pesticides
C. Polychlorinated Biphenyls (PCBs) in Water and Wastewater, Method for
D. Trihalomethanes
E. Volatile Chlorinated Organic Compounds in Water and Wastewaters,

---

[1] EPA Methods, March, 1979. See the full title of the Government publication in footnote 2 of TABLE A. Method numbers are those in the Government publication as noted in TABLE A.

[2] Methods for Uranium available in a recent EPA publication which is not yet referred to in 40 C.F.R. Part 141. See the full title of the Goverment publication in TABLE A, Footnote 8.

[3] EPA Methods, 1974. See the full title of the Government publication in footnote 1 of TABLE A. Page references are to the location of the methods in the Government publication as noted in TABLE A.

[4] EPA Interim Methods, September, 1978. See the full title of the Government publication in footnote 3 of TABLE A. Page references are to the location of the methods in the Government publication as noted in TABLES A, B and C.

[5] U.S. Geological Survey water method. See the full title of the Government publication in footnote 5 of TABLE C. Page reference is to the location of the method in the Government publication as noted in Table C.

INTRODUCTION

This "Supplement to the Fifteenth Edition of *Standard Methods for the Examination of Water and Wastewater*" (Supplement) presents selected analytical methods for which no equivalent methods are found in the Fifteenth Edition of *Standard Methods for the Examination of Water and Wastewater (Standard Methods)*, and which may be of use in complying with certain requirements of the National Pollution Discharge Elimination System (NPDES) regulations and the National Interim Primary Drinking Water Regulations promulgated by the U.S. Environmental Protection Agency (EPA).

EPA's regulations which approve and cite analytical water methods were promulgated prior to the publication of the Fifteenth Edition of *Standard Methods*, and therefore cite methods in the Fourteenth Edition. Many methods of analysis not included in the Fourteenth Edition, but required by EPA's regulations, have now been included in the Fifteenth Edition of *Standard Methods*, and it is expected that these methods will be approved and cited by EPA in the next revision of these regulations.

This Supplement provides information on analytical methods cited in regulations contained in Title 40 of the Code of Federal Regulations (C.F.R., July 1, 1980 ed.), primarily Part 136 (the NPDES regulations approving water methods) and Part 141 (the safe drinking water regulations). One of the several tables prepared by the Editors of the Supplement presents a listing of all the Federal regulations of EPA and other Federal agencies as of December 31, 1980 which refer to water methods.

Many of these regulations cite EPA's Table I.–List of Approved Test Procedures, set forth at 40 C.F.R. §136.3, which cites approved water methods for over 115 parameters, pollutants, and characteristics. The entire text of this basic regulation is presented in the Supplement.

The Government methods published by EPA which are included in the Supplement have not been subjected to the rigorous consensus approval procedures used to develop the standards methods contained in the Fifteenth Edition of *Standard Methods*. These Government methods are being presented without endorsement or sanction by the sponsors of *Standard Methods* as a service to the analyst. In addition, the publication of these supplemental methods should not be construed as approval of trade names cited by EPA or implied disapproval of comparable unlisted products. The mention of trade names or commercial products in the Supplement or the original EPA publications is for illustration purposes and does not constitute endorsement or recommendation for use by EPA or other agencies of the U.S. Government or by *Standard Methods*.

The methods presented in the Supplement include metals, inorganic nonmetals, organic compounds, and radioactive metals. Table I is the primary reference source for methods to be used in the analysis for pollutants. The term "pollutants" is also used to define the naturally occurring constituents of drinking water. Table I as presented in the Supplement does not include any of the changes in a proposed rule issued by EPA in the Federal Register on December 3, 1979 (44 Fed. Reg. 69464-575, as corrected by 44 Fed. Reg. 75029-52 (Dec. 18, 1979)), because those regulations have not yet been promulgated as a final rule. When EPA promulgates a revised version of Table I in Part 136, it will approve and cite methods in the Fifteenth Edition.

The Editors of the Supplement have prepared five tables, Tables A-E, to assist analysts in understanding EPA's TABLE I, the Federal regulations of all agencies, and the correlation between the Fourteenth and Fifteenth Editions.

It should be noted that there are several stages of method "approval". The official source of approved methods is the C.F.R., but there are appreciable delays in incorporating changes into the C.F.R. Moreover, once the final revised regulations are published in the Federal Register, it takes some time before the changes are incorporated in the C.F.R. Consequently, to meet new analytical demands, methods may be temporarily acceptable as recommended, proposed, interim, or as part of a proposed rule not yet incorporated into the current issue of the C.F.R. The status of a new method for reporting purposes is best determined by consultation with the agency in your State exercising primacy in the enforcement of State or Federal regulations.

The sponsors of *Standard Methods* wish to acknowledge the efforts of the Consulting Editor of the Supplement, Robert E. Mittendorff, Esq., for his thorough research of Federal regulations and Government water methods, and preparation of the various tables. Mr. Mittendorff is an attorney in Washington, D.C. who previously served in the Office of General Counsel of EPA. The sponsors also wish to recognize the diligent efforts of the Joint Editorial Board for *Standard Methods*—A. E. Greenberg, J. J. Connors, D. Jenkins and the Secretary, J. G. DeBoer, and most especially Mary Ann H. Franson, Managing Editor of the Fifteenth Edition.

The sponsors of *Standard Methods* are pleased to provide this Supplement with the Fifteenth Edition of *Standard Methods* so that analysts can benefit from a single source of analytical methods for the examination of water and wastewater.

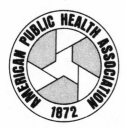 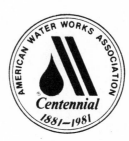 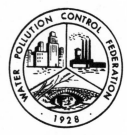

40 C.F.R. Part 136, § 136.3 (July 1, 1980 ed.)

TABLE I.—LIST OF APPROVED TEST PROCEDURES[1]

Parameter and units	Method	1974 EPA methods	14th ed. Standard Methods	References (page nos.) Pt. 31 1975 ASTM	References (page nos.) USGS methods[2]	Other approved methods
1. Acidity, as CaCO₃, milligrams per liter.	Electrometric end point (pH of 8.2) or phenolphthalein end point.	1	273(4d)	116	40	3(607)
2. Alkalinity, as CaCO₃, milligrams per liter.	Electrometric titration (only to pH 4.5) manual or automated, or equivalent automated methods.	3 5	278	111	41	3(607) —
3. Ammonia (as N), milligrams per liter.	Manual distillation[4] (at pH 9.5) followed by nesslerization, titration, electrode, automated phenolate.	159 165 168	410 412 616	237	116	3(614)
BACTERIA 4. Coliform (fecal)[5], number per 100 ml.	MPN;[6] membrane filter	—	922 937	—	7(45)	—
5. Coliform (fecal)[5] in presence of chlorine, number per 100 ml.	do.[6-8]	—	922	—	—	—
6. Coliform, (total),[5] number per 100 ml.	do.[6]	—	928, 937 916 928	—	7(35)	—
7. Coliform (total)[5] in presence of chlorine, number per 100 ml.	MPN;[6] membrane filter with enrichment.	—	916 933	—	—	—
8. Fecal streptococci,[5] number per 100 ml.	MPN;[6] membrane filter; plate count.	—	943 944 947	—	7(50)	—
9. Benzidine, milligrams per liter	Oxidation—colorimetric[9]	—	—	—	—	—
10. Biochemical oxygen demand, 5-d (BOD₅). milligrams per liter.	Winkler (Azide modification) or electrode method.	—	543	—	7(50)	10(17)
11. Bromide, milligrams per liter	Titrimetric, iodine-iodate	14	—	323	58	3(610)
12. Chemical oxygen demand (COD), milligrams per liter.	Dichromate reflux	20	550	472	124	10(17)
13. Chloride, milligrams per liter	Silver nitrate; mercuric nitrate; or automated colorimetric ferricyanide.	29 31	303 304 613	267 265	11(46)	3(615) 3(615)

No.	Parameter	Method					
14.	Chlorinated organic compounds (except pesticides), milligrams per liter.	Gas chromatography[12]	—	—	—	—	—
15.	Chlorine—total residual, milligrams per liter.	Iodometric titration, amperometric or starch-iodine end-point; DPD colorimetric or titrimetric methods (these last 2 are interim methods pending laboratory testing).	35	318, 322, 332, 329	278	—	—
16.	Color, platinum cobalt units or dominant wave length, hue, luminance, purity.	Colorimetric; spectrophotometric; or ADMI procedure.[13]	36, 39	64, 66	—	82	—
17.	Cyanide, total,[14] milligrams per liter	Distillation followed by silver nitrate titration or pyridine pyrazolone (or barbituric acid) colorimetric.	40	361	503	85	10(22)
18.	Cyanide amenable to chlorination, milligrams per liter.	do	49	376	505	—	—
19.	Dissolved oxygen, milligrams per liter.	Winkler (Azide modification) or electrode method.	51, 56	443, 450	368	126	3(609)
20.	Fluoride, milligrams per liter	Distillation[4] followed by ion electrode; SPADNS; or automated complexone.	65, 59, 61	389, 391, 393	307, 305	93	—
21.	Hardness—Total, as $CaCO_3$, milligrams per liter.	EDTA titration; automated colorimetric; or atomic absorption (sum of Ca and Mg as their respective carbonates)	68, 70	614, 202	161	94	3(617)
22.	Hydrogen ion (pH), pH units	Electrometric measurement	239	460	178	129	3(606)
23.	Kjeldahl nitrogen (as N), milligrams per liter.	Digestion and distillation followed by nesslerization, titration, or electrode; automated digestion automated phenolate.	175, 165, 182	437	—	122	3(612)
	METALS						
24.	Aluminum—Total, milligrams per liter.	Digestion[15] followed by atomic absorption[16] or by colorimetric (Eriochrome Cyanine R).	92	152, 171	—	11(19)	—
25.	Aluminum—Dissolved, milligrams per liter.	0.45 micron filtration[17] followed by referenced methods for total aluminum.	—	—	—	—	—
26.	Antimony—Total, milligrams per liter.	Digestion[15] followed by atomic absorption.[16]	94	—	—	—	—
27.	Antimony—Dissolved, milligrams per liter	0.45 micron filtration[17] followed by referenced method for total antimony.	—	—	—	—	—
28.	Arsenic—Total, milligrams per liter.	Digestion followed by silver diethyldithiocarbamate; or atomic absorption.[16][18]	9	285, 283	—	11(31)	—
29.	Arsenic—Dissolved, milligrams per liter.	0.45 micron filtration[17] followed by referenced method for total arsenic.	95	159	—	11(37)	—

TABLE I.—LIST OF APPROVED TEST PROCEDURES[1]—Continued

Parameter and units	Method	1974 EPA methods	14th ed. Standard Methods	Pt. 31 1975 ASTM	USGS methods[2]	Other approved methods
30. Barium—Total, milligrams per liter.	Digestion[15] followed by atomic absorption.[16]	97	152	—	52	—
31. Barium—Dissolved, milligrams per liter.	0.45 micron filtration[17] followed by referenced method for total barium.	—	—	—	—	—
32. Beryllium—Total, milligrams per liter.	Digestion[15] followed by atomic absorption[16] or by colorimetric (Aluminon).	99	152 / 177	—	53	—
33. Beryllium—Dissolved, milligrams per liter.	0.45 micron filtration[17] followed by referenced method for total beryllium.	—	—	—	—	—
34. Boron—Total, milligrams per liter.	Colorimetric (Curcumin)	13	287	—	—	—
35. Boron—Dissolved, milligrams per liter.	0.45 micron filtration[17] followed by referenced method for total boron.	—	—	—	—	—
36. Cadmium—Total, milligrams per liter.	Digestion[15] followed by atomic absorption[16] or by colorimetric (Dithizone).	101	148 / 182	345	62	3(619) / 10(37)
37. Cadmium—Dissolved, milligrams per liter.	0.45 micron filtration[17] followed by referenced method for total cadmium.	—	—	—	—	—
38. Calcium—Total, milligrams per liter.	Digestion[15] followed by absorption; or EDTA titration.	103	148 / 189	345	66	—
39. Calcium—Dissolved, milligrams per liter.	0.45 micron filtration[17] followed by referenced method for total calcium.	—	—	—	—	—
40. Chromium VI, milligrams per liter.	Extraction and atomic absorption; colorimetric (Diphenylcarbazide).	89, 105	192	—	76 / 75	—
41. Chromium VI—Dissolved, milligrams per liter.	0.45 micron filtration[17] followed by referenced method for chromium VI.	—	—	—	—	—
42. Chromium—Total, milligrams per liter.	Digestion[15] followed by atomic absorption[16] or by colorimetric (Diphenylcarbazide).	105	148 / 192	345 / 286	78 / 77	3(619)
43. Chromium—Dissolved, milligrams per liter.	0.45 micron filtration[17] followed by referenced method for total chromium.	—	—	—	—	—
44. Cobalt—Total, milligrams per liter.	Digestion[15] followed by atomic absorption.[16]	107	148	345	80	10(37)
45. Cobalt—Dissolved, milligrams per liter.	0.45 micron filtration[17] followed by referenced method for total cobalt.	—	—	—	—	—
46. Copper—Total, milligrams per liter.	Digestion[15] followed by atomic absorption[16] or by colorimetric (Neocuproine).	108	148 / 196	345 / 293	83	3(619) / 10(37)

No.	Parameter and method					
47.	Copper—Dissolved, milligrams per liter. 0.45 micron filtration[17] followed by referenced method for total copper.	—	—	—	—	—
48.	Gold—Total, milligrams per liter. Digestion[15] followed by atomic absorption.[19]	—	—	—	—	—
49.	Iridium—Total, milligrams per liter. Digestion[15] followed by atomic absorption.[19]	—	—	—	—	[3](619)
50.	Iron—Total, milligrams per liter. Digestion[15] followed by atomic absorption[16] or by colorimetric (Phenanthroline).	110	148	345	102	—
51.	Iron—Dissolved, milligrams per liter. 0.45 micron filtration[17] followed by referenced method for total iron.	—	208	326	—	—
52.	Lead—Total, milligrams per liter. Digestion[15] followed by atomic absorption[16] or by colorimetric (Dithizone)	112	148	345	105	[3](619)
53.	Lead—Dissolved, milligrams per liter. 0.45 micron filtration[17] followed by referenced method for total lead.	—	215	—	—	—
54.	Magnesium—Total, milligrams per liter. Digestion[15] followed by atomic absorption; or gravimetric.	114	148	345	109	[3](619)
55.	Magnesium—Dissolved, milligrams per liter. 0.45 micron filtration[17] followed by referenced method for total magnesium.	—	221	—	—	—
56.	Manganese—Total, milligrams per liter. Digestion[15] followed by atomic absorption[16] or by colorimetric (Persulfate or periodiate).	116	148	345	111	[3](619)
57.	Manganese—Dissolved, milligrams per liter. 0.45 micron filtration[17] followed by referenced method for total manganese.	—	225, 227	—	—	—
58.	Mercury—Total, milligrams per liter. Flameless atomic absorption.	118	156	338	[11](51)	—
59.	Mercury—Dissolved, milligrams per liter. 0.45 micron filtration[17] followed by referenced method for total mercury.	—	—	—	—	—
60.	Molybdenum—Total, milligrams per liter. Digestion[15] followed by atomic absorption.[16]	139	—	350	—	—
61.	Molybdenum—Dissolved, milligrams per liter. 0.45 micron filtration[17] followed by referenced method for total molybdenum.	—	—	—	—	—
62.	Nickel—Total, milligrams per liter. Digestion[15] followed by atomic absorption[16] or by colorimetric (Heptoxime).	141	148	345	115	—
63.	Nickel—Dissolved, milligrams per liter. 0.45 micron filtration[17] followed by referenced method for total nickel.	223	—	—	—	—
64.	Osmium—Total, milligrams per liter. Digestion[15] followed by atomic absorption.[19]	—	—	—	—	—
65.	Palladium—Total, milligrams per liter. Digestion[15] followed by atomic absorption.[19]	—	—	—	—	—
66.	Platinum—Total, milligrams per liter. Digestion[15] followed by atomic absorption.[19]	143	—	—	—	—
67.	Potassium—Total, milligrams per liter. Digestion[15] followed by atomic absorption, colorimetric (Cobaltinitrite), or by flame photometric.	—	235	403	134	[3](620)
68.	Potassium—Dissolved, milligrams per liter. 0.45 micron filtration[17] followed by referenced method for total potassium.	—	234	—	—	—

TABLE I.—LIST OF APPROVED TEST PROCEDURES[1]—Continued

Parameter and units	Method	1974 EPA methods	14th ed. standard methods	Pt. 31 1975 ASTM	USGS methods[2]	Other approved methods
69. Rhodium—Total, milligrams per liter.	Digestion[15] followed by atomic absorption.[19]	—	—	—	—	—
70. Ruthenium—Total, milligrams per liter.	Digestion[15] followed by atomic absorption.[19]	—	—	—	—	—
71. Selenium—Total, milligrams per liter.	Digestion[15] followed by atomic absorption.[19]	145	159	—	—	—
72. Selenium—Dissolved, milligrams per liter.	0.45 micron filtration[17] followed by reference method for total selenium.	—	—	—	—	—
73. Silica—Dissolved, milligrams per liter.	0.45 micron filtration[17] followed by colorimetric (Molybdosilicate).	274	487	398	139	—
74. Silver—Total,[20] milligrams per liter.	Digestion[15] followed by atomic absorption[16] or by colorimetric (Dithizone).	146	148 / 243	—	142	3(619) / 10(37)
75. Silver—Dissolved,[20] milligrams per liter.	0.45 micron filtration[17] followed by reference method for total silver.	—	—	—	—	—
76. Sodium—Total, milligrams per liter.	Digestion[15] followed by atomic absorption or by flame photometric.	147	250	403	143	3(621)
77. Sodium—Dissolved, milligrams per liter.	0.45 micron filtration[17] followed by reference method for total sodium.	—	—	—	—	—
78. Thallium—Total, milligrams per liter.	Digestion[15] followed by atomic absorption.[16]	149	—	—	—	—
79. Thallium—Dissolved, milligrams per liter.	0.45 micron filtration[17] followed by reference method for total thallium.	—	—	—	—	—
80. Tin—Total, milligrams per liter.	Digestion[15] followed by atomic absorption.[16]	150	—	—	11(65)	—
81. Tin—Dissolved, milligrams per liter.	0.45 micron filtration[17] followed by reference method for total tin.	—	—	—	—	—
82. Titanium—Total, milligrams per liter.	Digestion[15] followed by atomic absorption.[16]	151	—	—	—	—
83. Titanium—Dissolved, milligrams per liter.	0.45 micron filtration[17] followed by reference method for total titanium.	—	—	—	—	—
84. Vanadium—Total, milligrams per liter.	Digestion[15] followed by atomic absorption[16] or by colorimetric (Gallic acid).	153	152 / 260	441	11(67)	—
85. Vanadium—Dissolved, milligrams per liter.	0.45 micron filtration[17] followed by reference method for total vanadium.	—	—	—	—	—
86. Zinc—Total, milligrams per liter.	Digestion[15] followed by atomic absorption[16] or by colorimetric (Dithizone).	155	148 / 265	345	159	3(619) / 10(37)

No. & Constituent	Method	(1)	(2)	(3)	(4)	(5)
87. Zinc—Dissolved, milligrams per liter.	0.45 micron filtration[17] followed by referenced method for total zinc.	—	—	—	—	—
88. Nitrate (as N), milligrams per liter.	Cadmium reduction; brucine sulfate; automated cadmium or hydrazine reduction.[21]	201, 197, 207	423, 427, 620	358	119	[3](614), [10](28)
89. Nitrite (as N), milligrams per liter.	Manual or automated colorimetric (Diazotization).	215	434	—	121	—
90. Oil and grease, milligrams per liter.	Liquid-liquid extraction with trichloro-trifluoro-ethane-gravimetric.	229	515	—	—	—
91. Organic carbon; total (TOC), milligrams per liter.	Combustion—Infrared method.[22]	236	532	467	—	[23](4)
92. Organic nitrogen (as N), milligrams per liter.	Kjeldahl nitrogen minus ammonia nitrogen.	175, 159	437	—	122	[3](612, 614)
93. Orthophosphate (as P), milligrams per liter.	Manual or automated ascorbic acid reduction.	249, 256	481; 624	384	131	[3](621)
94. Pentachlorophenol, milligrams per liter.	Gas chromatography.[12]	—	—	—	—	—
95. Pesticides, milligrams per liter.	do.[12]	—	555	529	—	[23](24)
96. Phenols, milligrams per liter.	Distillation followed by Colorimetric (4AAP)	241	574	545	—	—
97. Phosphorus (elemental), milligrams per liter.	Gas chromatography.[24]	—	—	—	—	—
98. Phosphorus; total (as P), milligrams per liter.	Persulfate digestion followed by manual or automated ascorbic acid reduction.	249, 256	476, 481; 624	384	133	[3](621)
RADIOLOGICAL						
99. Alpha—Total, pCi per liter.	Proportional or scintillation counter.	—	648	591	[11], [25](75 + 78)	—
100. Alpha—Counting error, pCi per liter.	do.	—	648	594	[11](79)	—
101. Beta—Total, pCi per liter.	Proportional counter	—	648	601	[11], [25](75 + 78)	—
102. Beta—Counting error, pCi per liter.	do.	—	648	606	[11](79)	—
103. (a) Radium—Total, pCi per liter.	do.	—	661	661	[11](81)	—
(b) 226Ra, pCi per liter.	Scintillation counter.	—	667	—	—	—
RESIDUE						
104. Total, milligrams per liter.	Gravimetric, 103 to 105°C.	270	91	—	—	—
105. Total dissolved (filterable), milligrams per liter.	Glass fiber filtration, 180°C.	266	92	—	—	—
106. Total suspended residue.	Glass fiber filtration, 103 to 105°C., post-washing of residue.	268	94	—	—	[27](537)
107. Settleable, milliliters per liter or milligrams per liter.	Volumetric or gravimetric.	—	95	—	—	—
108. Total volatile, milligrams per liter.	Gravimetric, 550°C.	272	95	—	—	—

TABLE I.—LIST OF APPROVED TEST PROCEDURES[1]—Continued

Parameter and units	Method	References (page nos.)				
		1974 EPA methods	14th ed. standard methods	Pt. 31 1975 ASTM	USGS methods[2]	Other approved methods
109. Specific conductance, micromhos per centimeter at 25°C.	Wheatstone bridge conductimetry.	275	71	120	148	3(606)
110. Sulfate (as SO₄), milligrams per liter.	Gravimetric; turbidimetric; or automated colorimetric (barium chloranilate).	— 277 279	493 496	424 425	—	3(624) 3(623)
111. Sulfide (as S), milligrams per liter.	Titrimetric—Iodine for levels greater than 1 mg per liter; Methylene blue photometric.	284	505 503	—	154	—
112. Sulfite (as SO₃), milligrams per liter.	Titrimetric, iodine-iodate.	285	508	435	—	—
113. Surfactants, milligrams per liter.	Colorimetric (Methylene blue).	157	600	494	22(11)	—
114. Temperature, degrees C.	Calibrated glass or electrometric thermometer.	286	125	—	26(31)	—
115. Turbidity, NTU.	Nephelometric.	295	132	223	156	—

[1] Recommendations for sampling and preservation of samples according to parameter measured may be found in "Methods for Chemical Analysis of Water and Wastes, 1974" U.S. Environmental Protection Agency, table 2, pp. viii–xii.

[2] All page references for USGS methods, unless otherwise noted, are to Brown, E., Skougstad, M.W., and Fishman, M.J., "Methods for Collection and Analysis of Water Samples for Dissolved Minerals and Gases," U.S. Geological Survey Techniques of Water-Resources Inv., book 5, ch. Al. (1970).

[3] EPA comparable method may be found on indicated page of "Official Methods of Analysis of the Association of Official Analytical Chemists" methods manual, 12th ed. (1975).

[4] Manual distillation is not required if comparability data on representative effluent samples are on company file to show that this preliminary distillation step is not necessary; however, manual distillation will be required to resolve any controversies.

[5] The method used must be specified.

[6] The 5 tube MPN is used.

[7] Slack, K.V. and others, "Methods for Collection and Analysis of Aquatic Biological and Microbiological Samples: U.S. Geological Survey Techniques of Water-Resources Inv. book 5, ch. A4 (1973)."

[8] Since the membrane filter technique usually yields low and variable recovery from chlorinated wastewaters, the MPN method will be required to resolve any controversies.

[9] Adequately tested methods for benzidine are not available. Until approved methods are available, the following interim method can be used for the estimation of benzidine: (1) "Method for Benzidine and Its Salts in Wastewaters," available from Environmental Monitoring and Support Laboratory, U.S. Environmental Protection Agency, Cincinnati, Ohio 45268.

[10] American National Standard on Photographic Processing Effluents, Apr. 2, 1975. Available from ANSI, 1430 Broadway, New York, N.Y. 10018.

[11] Fishman, M.J. and Brown, Eugene, "Selected Methods of the U.S. Geological Survey for Analysis of Wastewaters," (1976) open-file report 76–177.

[12] Procedures for pentachlorophenol, chlorinated organic compounds, and pesticides can be obtained from the Environmental Monitoring and Support Laboratory, U.S. Environmental Protection Agency, Cincinnati, Ohio 45268.

[13] Color method (ADMI procedure) available from Environmental Monitoring and Support Laboratory, U.S. Environmental Protection Agency, Cincinnati, Ohio 45268.

[14] For samples suspected of having thiocyanate interference, magnesium chloride is used as the digestion catalyst. In the approved test procedure for cyanides, the recommended catalysts are replaced with 20 ml of a solution of 510 g/l magnesium chloride (MgCl₂·6H₂O). This substitution will eliminate thiocyanate interference for both total cyanide and cyanide amenable to chlorination measurements.

[15] For the determination of total metals the sample is not filtered before processing. Because vigorous digestion procedures may result in a loss of certain metals through precipitation, a less vigorous treatment is recommended as given on p. 83 (4.1.4) of "Methods for Chemical Analysis of Water and Wastes" (1974). In those instances where a more vigorous digestion is desired, the procedure on p. 82 (4.1.3) should be followed. For the measurement of the noble metal series (gold, iridium, osmium, palladium, platinum, rhodium and ruthenium), an aqua regia digestion is to be substituted as follows: Transfer a representative aliquot of the well-mixed sample to a Griffin beaker and add 3 ml of concentrated redistilled HNO₃. Place the beaker on a steam bath and evaporate to dryness. Cool the beaker and cautiously add a 5 ml portion of aqua regia. (Aqua regia is prepared immediately before use by carefully adding 3 volumes of concentrated HCl to one volume of concentrated HNO₃). Cover the beaker with a watch glass and return to the steam bath. Continue heating the covered beaker for 30 min. Remove cover and evaporate to dryness. Cool and take up the residue in a small quantity of 1:1 HCl. Wash down the beaker walls and wash glass with distilled water and filter the sample to remove silicates and other insoluble material that could clog the atomizer. Adjust the volume to some predetermined value based on the expected metal concentration. The sample is now ready for analysis.

[16] As the various furnace devices (flameless AA) are essentially atomic absorption techniques, they are considered to be approved test methods. Methods of standard addition are to be followed as noted in p. 78 of "Methods for Chemical Analysis of Water and Wastes," 1974.

[17] Dissolved metals are defined as those constituents which will pass through a 0.45 μm membrane filter. A prefiltration is permissible to free the sample from larger suspended solids. Filter the sample as soon as practical after collection using the first 50 to 100 ml to rinse the filter flask. (Glass or plastic filtering apparatus are recommended to avoid possible contamination.) Discard the portion used to rinse the flask and collect the required volume of filtrate. Acidify the filtrate with 1:1 redistilled HNO₃ to a pH of 2. Normally, 3 ml of (1:1) acid per liter should be sufficient to preserve the samples.

[18] See "Atomic Absorption Newsletter," vol. 13, 75 (1974). Available from Perkin-Elmer Corp., Main Ave., Norwalk, Conn. 06852.

[19] Method available from Environmental Monitoring and Support Laboratory, U.S. Environmental Protection Agency, Cincinnati, Ohio 45268.

[20] Recommended methods for the analysis of silver in industrial wastewaters at concentrations of 1 mg/l and above are inadequate where silver exists as an inorganic halide. Silver halides such as the bromide and chloride are relatively insoluble in reagents such as nitric acid but are readily soluble in an aqueous buffer of sodium thiosulfate and sodium hydroxide to a pH of 12. Therefore, for levels of silver above 1 mg/l 20 ml of sample should be diluted to 100 ml by adding 40 ml each of 2M Na₂S₂O₃ and 2M NaOH. Standards should be prepared in the same manner. For levels of silver below 1 mg/l the recommended method is satisfactory.

[21] An automated hydrazine reduction method is available from the Environmental Monitoring and Support Laboratory, U.S. Environmental Protection Agency, Cincinnati, Ohio 45268.

[22] A number of such systems manufactured by various companies are considered to be comparable in their performance. In addition, another technique, based on combustion-methane detection is also acceptable.

[23] Goeritz, D., Brown, E., "Methods for Analysis of Organic Substances in Water": U.S. Geological Survey Techniques of Water-Resources Inv., book 5, ch. A3 (1972).

[24] R.F. Addison and R.G. Ackman, "Direct Determination of Elemental Phosphorus by Gas-Liquid Chromatography," "Journal of Chromatography," vol. 47, No. 3, pp. 421–426, 1970.

[25] The method found on p. 75 measures only the dissolved portion while the method on p. 78 measures only suspended. Therefore, the 2 results must be added together to obtain "total."

[26] Stevens, H.H., Ficke, J.F., and Smoot, G.F., "Water Temperature—Influential Factors, Field Measurement and Data Presentation: U.S. Geological Survey Techniques of Water Resources Inv., book 1 (1975)."

[27] "Standard Methods for the Examination of Water and Wastewater, 13th Edition, (1971).

[38 FR 28758. Oct. 16, 1973, as amended at 41 FR 52781, Dec. 1, 1976; 42 FR 3306, Jan. 18, 1977; 42 FR 37205, July 20, 1977]

TABLE A. LISTING OF PARAMETERS AND APPROVED GOVERNMENT WATER METHODS NOT CONTAINED IN STANDARDS METHODS FOR THE EXAMINATION OF WATER AND WASTEWATER

Environmental Protection Agency Regulations Approving and Citing Methods	Parameter or Pollutant (Reference in EPA Table I. or Regulations)	Method (Description from EPA List)	Government Method (Page or method reference, and footnotes to § 136.3 as applicable)	Supplement (15th ed.) (Page reference to this text)
NPDES Wastewater Discharge Regulations. (Parameters listed in EPA's Guidelines Establishing Test Procedures, 40 C.F.R. Part 136, § 136.3, Table I-List of Approved Test Procedures).				
	9. Benzidine	Oxidation-colorimetric	1[3]	S48
	11. Bromide	Titrimetric, iodine—iodate	14[1]	S44
	14. Chlorinated organic compounds (except pesticides)	Gas chromatography	See Table B	S14
	65. Palladium-Total	Digestion/atomic absorption[4]	Method 253.1 or 253.2[2]	S27 S28
	94. Pentachlorophenol	Gas chromatography	140[3]	S50
	95. Pesticides	Gas chromatography	See Table C	S15
	97. Phosphorous (elemental)	Gas chromatography	Footnote 24	—
	— Metals, Total	Digestion followed by atomic absorption[4]	Footnotes 15 and 16	—[6]
	— Metals, Dissolved	Micron filtration[5]	Footnote 17	—[7]

National Interim Primary Drinking Water Regulations (Methods listed in 40 C.F.R. §§ 141.21–.25, .30, and .41.)			
Trihalomethanes in Drinking Water (§ 141.30(e)(2))	Liquid/Liquid Extraction Method	40 C.F.R. Part 141, Appendix C, Part II (44 Fed. Reg. 68624, 68683–89 as amended by 45 Fed. Reg. 15542–45, March 11, 1980.)	S92
Maximum Trihalomethanes (§ 141.30)	Determination of Maximum Trihalomethane Potential (MTP)	40 C.F.R. Part 141, Appendix C, Part III (July 1, 1980 ed.)	S101
Uranium (§ 141.25 (a)(7))	Radiochemical	Method 908.0, 96[8]	S32
Uranium (§ 141.25 (a)(7))	Fluorometric	Method 908.1, 103[8]	S36

[1] "Methods for Chemical Analysis of Water and Wastes, 1974," U.S. Environmental Protection Agency, Environmental Monitoring and Support Laboratory (EMSL), (EPA—625/6-74-003a); (referred to herein as "EPA Methods, 1974").

[2] "Methods for Chemical Analysis of Water and Wastes, March, 1979" U.S. Environmental Protection Agency, Environmental Monitoring and Support Laboratory (EMSL), (EPA —600/4-79-020); (referred to herein as "EPA Methods, March, 1979").

[3] "Methods for Benzidine, Chlorinated Organic Compounds, Pentachlorophenol and Pesticides in Water and Wastewater" (INTERIM, Pending Issuance of Methods for Organic Analysis of Water and Wastes, September 1978), U.S. Environmental Protection Agency, Environmental Monitoring and Support Laboratory (EMSL); (referred to herein as "EPA Interim Methods, September, 1978").

[4] Digestion (with reference to EPA Table I., text of footnote 15) followed by atomic absorption (with reference to EPA Table I., text of footnote 16).

[5] 0.45 Micro filtration (with reference to EPA Table I., footnote 17) followed by referenced method for total amount of same metal.

[6] The 14th edition did not include methods for total concentrations of the following metals, which are included in the 15th edition: Parameter 26, Antimony; 48, Gold; 49, Iridium; 60, Molybdenum; 64, Osmium; 66, Platinum; 69, Rhodium; 70, Ruthenium; 78, Thallium; 80, Tin; and 82, Titanium. See TABLE D of this Supplement for references to the methods contained in the 15th edition.

[7] The method for finding the amount of dissolved metal is simply 0.45 micron filtration followed by the method for the total metal. See Section 302A of the 15th edition and the methods of the 15th edition for dissolved metals referred to in TABLE D of this Supplement.

[8] Methods for Uranium are available in a recent EPA publication which is not yet referred to in 40 C.F.R. Part 141, "Prescribed Procedures for Measurement of Radioactivity in Drinking Water." Environmental Monitoring and Support Laboratory, Environmental Protection Agency, EPA-600/4-80-032, August, 1980. These methods have not yet been officially approved and cited by EPA in the Part 141 regulations; however, they represent two new Government methods for Uranium.

TABLE B. APPROVED METHODS FOR PARAMETER 14., CHLORINATED ORGANIC COMPOUNDS

(Listing of Chlorinated Organic Compounds and approval of the Methods in Standard Methods for the Examination of Water and Wastewater or EPA Methods).[1]

Chlorinated Organic Compounds	EPA Approval of Method 509 A, Fourteenth Edition, Standard Methods (Page reference)	Government Method (Page reference)	Supplement (Page reference to Government Method)
Heptachloro epoxide	555	—	—
Benzylchloride, Carbon tetrachloride, Chlorobenzene, Chloroform, Epichlorohydrin, Methylene chloride, 1,1,2,2-Tetrachloroethane, Tetrachloroethylene, 1,2,4-Trichloro-benzene	—	130[1]	S102
Polychlorinated biphenyls (PCB's) including the following chlorinated biphenyls (Aroclors): PCB-1016, PCB-1221, PCB-1232, PCB-1242, PCB-1248, PCB-1254, and PCB-1260	—	43[1]	S78

[1] In the Foreword of its publication of methods entitled "Methods for Benzidine, Chlorinated Organic Compounds, Pentachlorophenol and Pesticides in Water and Wastewater" (INTERIM, Pending Issuance of Methods for Organic Analysis of Water and Wastes, September 1978), U.S. Environmental Protection Agency, Environmental Monitoring and Support Laboratory (EMSL), EPA states that the referenced methods are to be used for the NPDES Permits Program. The publication includes an index to page references indicating approval of Method 509 A. of the Fourteenth Edition of Standard Methods (1974), pages 555 *et seq.*, for certain compounds. Page references are to the Government methods included in the publication described above. The basis for EMSL's adoption of these methods for NPDES purposes is established in 40 C.F.R. Part 136, Guidelines Establishing Test Procedures, Table I-List of Approved Test Procedures, which states in Footnote 12 that approved methods are available from EMSL.

TABLE C. APPROVED METHODS FOR PARAMETER 95., PESTICIDES

(Listing of Pesticides and approval of the Methods in Standard Methods for the Examination of Water and Wastewater or EPA and other Government Methods).[2]

Pesticides	EPA Approval Method 509 A., Fourteenth Edition, Standard Methods (Page reference)	Government Method (Page reference)	Supplement (Page reference to Government Method)
Aldrin, BHC, Captan, Chlordane, DDD, DDE, DDT, Dichloran, Endosulfan, Endrin, Heptachlor, Lindane, Methoxychlor, Mirex, PCNB, Strobane, and Toxaphene	555[1]	7[2]	—
Dieldrin and Trifluraline	—[3]	7[2]	—
Malathion, Parathion methyl, and Parathion ethyl	555[3]	25[2]	S51
Azinphos methyl, Demeton-O, Diazinon, Disulfoton	—	25[2]	S51
Ametryn, Atraton, Atrazine, Prometon, Prometryn, Propazine, Secbumeton, Simazine and Terbuthylazine	—	83[2]	S68
Aminocarb, Carbaryl, Methiocarb, Mexacarbate, and Proporur	—	94[2]	S60
Barban, Chlorpropham, Diuron, Fenuron, Fenuron-TCA, Linuron, Monuron, Monuron-TCA, Neburon, Propham, Siduron, and Swep	—	104[2]	S64
2,4-D, Dicamba, Silvex, and 2,4,5-T	—[4]	115[2]	—
Carbophenothion, Dichlorofenthion, Dioxathion, Ethion, and Isodrin	—	30[5]	S73
Dicofol and Perthane[6]	—	—	—

[1] See Method 509A, p. 493 of the 15th Edition for an equivalent method.

[2] In the Foreword of its publication of methods entitled "Methods for Benzidine, Chlorinated Organic Compounds, Pentachlorophenol and Pesticides in Water and Wastewater" (INTERIM, Pending Issuance of Methods for Organic Analysis of Water and Wastes, September 1978), U.S. Environmental Protection Agency, Environmental Monitoring and Support Laboratory (EMSL), EPA states that the referenced methods are to be used for the NPDES Permits Program. The publication includes an index to page references indicating approval of Method 509A. of the Fourteenth Edition of Standard Methods (1974), pages 555 *et seq.*, for certain compounds and pesticides as illustrated in the above table. Page references are to the Government methods included in the publication described above. The basis for EMSL's adoption of these methods for NPDES purposes is established in 40 C.F.R. Part 136, Guidelines Establishing Test Procedures, Table I-List of Approved Test Procedures, which states in Footnote 12 that approved methods are available from EMSL.

[3] These pesticides may be determined by Method 509A, p. 493, Standard Methods, 15th Edition under favorable circumstances. Analyst must confirm. The EPA method referred to for Dieldrin and Trifluraline is substantially identical to Method 509A and is not included in the Supplement.

[4] These pesticides may be determined by Method 509B, p. 504, Standard Methods, 15th Edition.

[5] "Methods for Analysis of Organic Substances in Water" by D.F. Goerlitz and Eugene Brown, U.S. Geological Survey, Techniques of Water-Resources Investigations, Book 5, Chapter A3 (1972).

[6] See 40 C.F.R. Part 136, Table I., Parameter 95. Pesticides, reference to p. 529 of ASTM (1975).

TABLE D. CORRELATION BETWEEN APPROVED METHODS CONTAINED IN THE FOURTEENTH EDITION (1976) OF STANDARD METHODS FOR THE EXAMINATION OF WATER AND WASTEWATER CITED IN EPA REGULATIONS AND EQUIVALENT METHODS CONTAINED IN THE FIFTEENTH EDITION (1981)

Government Regulation	Constituent or Parameter	Fourteenth Edition		Fifteenth Edition	
		Method	Page	Method	Page[1]
40 C.F.R. Part 136, Guidelines Establishing Test Procedures, § 136.3 Table I.— List of Approved Test Procedures	NPDES WASTEWATER DISCHARGE REGULATIONS				
	1 Acidity	402(4d)	273	402(4d)	249
	2 Alkalinity	403	278	403	253
	3 Ammonia	418A+B; 604	410, 412, 616	417A+B; E	355, 356, 363
	Bacteria:				
	4 Coliform (fecal)	908C; 909C	922, 937	908C; 909C	801, 814
	5 Coliform (fecal) (chlorine)	908C; 909; 909C	922, 928, 937	908C; 909; 909C	801, 806, 814
	6 Coliform (total)	908A; 909A	916, 928	908A; 909A	796, 806
	7 Coliform (total) (chlorine)	908A; 909A.5c	916, 933	908A; 909A.5c	796, 810
	8 Fecal streptococci	910A; B; C	943, 944, 947	910A; B; C	819, 821, 822
	9 Benzidine	—	—	—	S48
	10 Biochemical oxygen demand	507	543	507	483
	11 Bromide	—	—	—	S44
	12 Chemical oxygen demand	508	550	508	489
	13 Chloride	408A; B; 602	303, 304, 613	407A; B; D	270, 271, 275
	14 Chlorinated organic compounds (except pesticides)	—	—	—	See Table B
	15 Chlorine, total residual	409B; C; E; F	318, 322, 329, 332	408B; C; D; E	283, 286, 289, 292
	16 Color	204A; B	64, 66	204A; B	61, 63
	17 Cyanide (total)	413B+(C; D)	367, 369, 370	412B+(C; D)	317, 319, 320
	18 Cyanide (chlorination)	413F	376	412F	324
	19 Dissolved oxygen	422B; F	443, 450	421B; F	390, 395
	20 Fluoride	414A; B; C; 603	389, 391, 393, 614	413A; B; C; E	334, 335, 337, 340
	21 Hardness	309B	202	303A+314A	152, 195

		424 / 421	460 / 437	423 / 420	402 / 383
22	Hydrogen ion (pH)				
23	Kjeldahl nitrogen (N)				
	Metal parameters:				
24, 25	Aluminum, total and dissolved[2]	301A.IV; 302B	152, 171	303C; 306B	157, 169
26, 27	Antimony, total and dissolved[2]	—	—	303A	152
28, 29	Arsenic, total and dissolved[2]	301A.VII; 404A	159, 283, 285	303E; 307B	160, 174
30, 31	Barium, total and dissolved[2]	301A.IV	152	303C	157
32, 33	Beryllium, total and dissolved[2]	301A.IV; 304B	152, 177	303C; 309B	157, 178
34, 35	Boron, total and dissolved[2]	405A	287	404A	257
36, 37	Cadmium, total and dissolved[2]	301A.II; 305C	148, 182	303A; 310B	152, 180
38, 39	Calcium, total and dissolved[2]	301A.II; 306C	148, 189	303A; 311C	152, 185
40, 41	Chromium VI, total and dissolved[2]	307B	192	312B	187
42, 43	Chromium, total and dissolved[2]	301A.II; 307B	148, 192	303A; 312B	152, 187
44, 45	Cobalt, total and dissolved[2]	301A.II	148	303A	152
46, 47	Copper, total and dissolved[2]	301A.II; 308B	148, 196	303A; 313B	152, 191
48	Gold, total	—	—	303A	152
49	Iridium, total	—	—	303A	152
50, 51	Iron, total and dissolved[2]	301A.II; 310A	148, 208	303A; 315B	152, 201
52, 53	Lead, total and dissolved[2]	301A.II; 311B	148, 215	303A; 316B	152, 207
54, 55	Magnesium, total and dissolved[2]	301A.II; 313A	148, 221	303A+318B	152, 211
56, 57	Manganese, total and dissolved[2]	301A.II; 314B; C[3]	148, 225, 227[3]	303A+319B	152, 214
58, 59	Mercury, total and dissolved[2]	301A.VI	156	303F	164
60, 61	Molybdenum, total and dissolved[2]			303C	157
62, 63	Nickel, total and dissolved[2]	301A.II	148	303A	152
64	Osmium, total	—	—	303C	157
65	Palladium, total	—	—	—	S27, S28
66	Platinum, total	—	—	303A	152
67, 68	Potassium, total and dissolved[2]	317A; B[3]	234, 235[3]	303A; 322B	152, 221
69	Rhodium, total	—	—	303A	152
70	Ruthenium, total			303A	152
71, 72	Selenium, total and dissolved[2]	301A.VII	159	303E	160
73	Silica, dissolved	426B	487	425C	429

TABLE D. CORRELATION OF APPROVED METHODS CONTAINED IN THE FOURTEENTH EDITION (1976) OF STANDARD METHODS FOR THE EXAMINATION OF WATER AND WASTEWATER AS REFERENCED IN EPA REGULATIONS AND OF EQUIVALENT METHODS IN THE FIFTEENTH EDITION (1981)—Continued

Government Regulation	Constituent or Parameter	Fourteenth Edition Method	Fourteenth Edition Page	Fifteenth Edition Method	Fifteenth Edition Page[1]
74, 75	Silver, total and dissolved[2]	301A.II; 319B	148, 243	303A; 324B	152, 227
76, 77	Sodium, total and dissolved[2]	320A	250	303A; 325B	152, 231
78, 79	Thallium, total and dissolved[2]	—	—	303A	152
80, 81	Tin, total and dissolved[2]	—	—	303A	152
82, 83	Titanium, total and dissolved[2]	—	—	303C	157
84, 85	Vanadium, total and dissolved[2]	301A.IV; 322B	152, 260	303C; 327B	157, 237
86, 87	Zinc, total and dissolved[2]	301A.II; 323C	148, 265	303A; 328C	152, 242
88	Nitrate (as N)	419C; D[3]; 605	423, 427[3], 620	418C; F	370, 376
89	Nitrite (as N)	420	434	419	380
90	Oil and grease	502A	515	503A	461
91	Organic carbon	505	532	505	471
92	Organic nitrogen (as N)	421	437	420A	383
93	Orthophosphate (as P)	425F; 606	481, 624	424F; G	420, 422
94	Pentachlorophenol	—	—	—	S50
95	Pesticides (See Table C)	509A	555	509A	493
96	Phenols	510A+B	576, 577	510A+B	509, 510
97	Phosphorus, elemental	—	—	—	—
98	Phosphorus, total (as P)	425F; 606	481, 624	424F; G	420, 422
	Radiological parameters:				
99	Alpha, total	703	648	703	574
100	Alpha, counting error	703	648	703	574
101	Beta, total	703	648	703	574
102	Beta, counting error	703	648	703	574
103	Radium, total	705; 706	661, 667	705, 706	585, 590
	Residue parameters:				
104	Total	208A	91	209A	92
105	Total dissolved	208B	92	209B	93
106	Total suspended residue	208D; 224C[4]	94, 537[4]	209D	94

107	Settleable	208F	95	209F	96
108	Total volatile	208E	95	209E	95
109	Specific conductance	205	71	205	70
110	Sulfate (as SO_4)	427A; C	493, 496	426A; C	436, 439
111	Sulfide (as S)	428C; D	503, 505	427C; D	447, 448
112	Sulfite (as SO_3)	429	508	428	451
113	Surfactants	512A	600	512A	530
114	Temperature	212	125	212	124
115	Turbidity, NTU	214A	132	214A	132

SAFE DRINKING WATER REGULATIONS

40 C.F.R. Part 141, National Interim Primary Drinking Water Regulations Subpart C—Monitoring and Analytical Requirements

40 C.F.R. §141.21 Microbiological contaminant sampling and analytical requirements

141.21 (a)	Coliform bacteria	908A; D, Table 908:I; 909A	916, 923, 928	908A; D, Table 908:I; 909A	796, 802, 806
141.21 (h)	Chlorine (residual)	114G[5]	129[5]	408D	289

TABLE D. CORRELATION OF APPROVED METHODS CONTAINED IN THE FOURTEENTH EDITION (1976) OF STANDARD METHODS FOR THE EXAMINATION OF WATER AND WASTEWATER AS REFERENCED IN EPA REGULATIONS AND OF EQUIVALENT METHODS IN THE FIFTEENTH EDITION (1981)—Continued

Government Regulation	Constituent or Parameter	Fourteenth Edition		Fifteenth Edition	
		Method	Page	Method	Page[1]
40 C.F.R. §141.22 Turbidity sampling and analytical requirements 141.22 (a)	Turbidity	214A	132	214A	132'
40 C.F.R. §141.23 Inorganic chemical sampling and analytical requirements 141.23 (f)	1 Arsenic	301A.VII; 404A+B.4	159, 283, 285	303E; 307B+C.4	160, 174, 176
	2 Barium	301A.IV	152	303C	157
	3 Cadmium	301A.II; III	148, 151	303A; B	152, 156
	4 Chromium	301A.II; III	148, 151	303A; B	152, 156
	5 Lead	301A.II; III	148, 151	303A; B	152, 156
	6 Mercury	301A.VI	156	303F	164
	7 Nitrate	419C; D; 605	423, 427, 620	418C, F	370, 376
	8 Selenium	301A.VII	159	303E	160
	9 Silver	301A.II	148	303A	152
	10 Fluoride	414A+C; B; 603	389, 393, 391, 614	413A+C; B; E	334, 337, 335, 340
40 C.F.R. §141.24 Organic chemicals					

other than total trihalomethanes, sampling and analytical requirements				
141.24 (e) Chlorinated hydrocarbons[6]	509A	555	509A	493
141.24 (f) Chlorophenoxys[7]	509B	565	509B	504
40 C.F.R. §141.25 Analytical Methods for Radioactivity				
141.25 (a) 1 Gross alpha and beta	302[5]	598[5]	703	574
2 Total radium	304[5]	611[5]	705	585
3 Radium 226	305[5]	617[5]	706	590
4 Strontium 89, 90	303[5]	604[5]	704	579
5 Tritium	306[5]	629[5]	708	603
6 Cesium-134	—	—	709	605[8]
7 Uranium	—	—	—	S32, S36
40 C.F.R. §141.30 Total trihalomethanes sampling, analytical and other requirements				
141.30 (e)(1) Trihalomethanes in Drinking Waters by the Purge and Trap Method	—	—	514	538
141.30 (e)(2) and Appendix C, Part II Trihalomethanes in Drinking Waters by Liquid/Liquid Extraction Method	—	—	—	S92

Table D. Correlation of Approved Methods Contained in the Fourteenth Edition (1976) of Standard Methods for the Examination of Water and Wastewater as Referenced in EPA Regulations and of Equivalent Methods in the Fifteenth Edition (1981)—Continued

Government Regulation	Constituent or Parameter	Fourteenth Edition		Fifteenth Edition	
		Method	Page	Method	Page[1]
141.30 (e)(2) and Appendix C, Part III	Maximum Total Trihalomethane Potential (MTP)[9]	—	—	—	S101
40 C.F.R. §141.41 Special monitoring for sodium	Sodium	320A	250	325B	231
40 C.F.R. §141.42 Special monitoring for corrosivity characteristics 141.42 (c)	1 Langelier Index	203	61	203	57
	2 Aggressive Index	—	—	—	—
	3 Total filtrable residue	208B	92	209B	93'
	4 Temperature	212	125	212	124
	5 Calcium hardness	309B	202	314B	195
	6 Alkalinity	403	278	403	253
	7 pH	424	460	423	402
	8 Chloride	408C	306	407C	273
	9 Sulfate	427C, 156C[4]	496, 334[4]	426C	439

[1] Page numbers preceded by "S" denote pages in this Supplement to "Standard Methods", 15th edition.

[2] For dissolved form of metal, filter sample according to Section 302A, 15th edition, before analyzing by referenced methods. This is essentially equivalent to the procedure given in footnote 17 of EPA's TABLE I.—List of approved test procedures, which appears in this Supplement at p. S4.

[3] Method not included in the 15th edition.

[4] Standard Methods for the Examination of Water and Wastewater, Thirteenth Edition (1971). The water method in the Fourteenth Edition for this parameter is also cited and approved by EPA.

[5] The referenced method is contained in the Thirteenth Edition of Standard Methods (1971). Although not yet officially approved for use, EPA intends to update the references in the regulations to those contained in the Fifteenth Edition or to those in the Fourteenth Edition (1976) which follow: Chlorine (residual)—Methods 409 E. and F., Gross Alpha and Beta—Method 703; Total Radium—Method 705; Radium-226—Method 706; Strontium 89, 90—Method 704; Tritium—Method 707.

[6] EPA lists the Chlorinated hydrocarbons in 40 C.F.R. § 141.12(a) to include Endrin, Lindane, Methoxychlor, and Toxaphene.

[7] EPA lists the Chlorophenoxys in 40 C.F.R. § 141.12(b) to include 2,4-D (2,4-Dichlorophenoxyacetic acid), 2,4,5-TP (Trichlorophenoxypropionic acid), Silvex.

[8] The method in the 15th edition covers both Cesium-134 and Cesium-137. A new method for radioactive Cesium developed by EPA, but not yet approved in its regulations, is substantially similar to the cited method in the 15th edition. See Method 901.0, p. 15 in the publication referred to in TABLE A, footnote 8 of this Supplement.

[9] EPA defines Total trihalomethanes in 40 C.F.R. § 141.12(c) as the sum of the concentrations of bromodichloromethane, dibromochloromethane, tribromomethane (bromoform) and trichloromethane (chloroform).

TABLE E. FEDERAL REGULATIONS REFERRING TO WATER METHODS

A. *Guidelines Establishing Test Procedures For the Analysis of Pollutants,* 40 C.F.R. Part 136 (July 1, 1980 ed.) (Environmental Protection Agency) including:
   (1.) Identification of test procedures.
        40 C.F.R. § 136.3
   (2.) TABLE I.—List of approved test procedures.
        40 C.F.R. § 136.3, TABLE I.[1]
B. *National Pollutant Discharge Elimination System* (Consolidated Permit Regulations) 40 C.F.R. Parts 122 and 125 (July 1, 1980 ed.) (Environmental Protection Agency)
   (1.) Monitoring and records.
        40 C.F.R. § 122.7(j)
   (2.) Requirements for recording and reporting of monitoring results.
        40 C.F.R. § 122.11
   (3.) Subpart D—Additional Requirements for National Pollutant Discharge Elimination System Programs under the Clean Water Act.
        40 C.F.R. § 122.51 through § 122.53(d); and § 122.60 through § 122.63
   (4.) Appendix D to Part 122-NPDES Permit Application Testing Requirements (§ 122.53)
        40 C.F.R. Part 122, Appendix D, Tables I-V
   (5.) Part 125, Subpart G—Criteria for Modifying the Secondary Treatment Requirement Under Section 301(h) of the Clean Water Act; Establishment of a monitoring system.
        40 C.F.R. § 125.62
C. *Regulations Related to the NPDES Program*
   (1.) Toxic Pollutant Effluent Standards.
        40 C.F.R. Part 129 (July 1, 1980 ed.) (Environmental Protection Agency)
        (a.) Aldrin/Dieldrin
             40 C.F.R. § 129.100
        (b.) DDT/DDD and DDE
             40 C.F.R. § 129.101
        (c.) Endrin
             40 C.F.R. § 129.102
        (d.) Toxaphene
             40 C.F.R. § 129.103
        (e.) Benzidine
             40 C.F.R. § 129.104
        (f.) Polychlorinated Biphenyls (PCBs)
             40 C.F.R. § 129.105
   (2.) Secondary Treatment Information.
        40 C.F.R. Part 133 (July 1, 1980 ed.) (Environmental Protection Agency
D. *Regulations of Other Federal Programs Adopting the Guidelines Establishing Test Procedures*
   (1.) Marine Sanitation Device Standard.
        40 C.F.R. Part 140 (July 1, 1980 ed.) (Environmental Protection Agency)
   (2.) Marine Sanitation Devices.
        33 C.F.R. Part 159 (July 1, 1980 ed.) (Department of Transportation, United States Coast Guard)
        Sewage processing test and other related tests.
        33 C.F.R. § 159.121 through § 159.127
   (3.) Subchapter B, Initial Program Regulations, Part 715—General Performance Standards and Part 717—Underground Mining General Performance Standards; 30 C.F.R. Parts 715 and 717.
        (July 1, 1980 ed.) (Department of Interior, Office of Surface Mining Reclamation and Enforcement ("OSM"))

TABLE E.   FEDERAL REGULATIONS REFERRING TO WATER METHODS—*Continued*

    (a.) Protection of the hydrologic system.
        30 C.F.R. § 715.17(a) through (d)
    (b.) Protection of the hydrologic system.
        30 C.F.R. § 717.17(a) through (d)
(4.) Subchapter G, Surface Coal Mining and Reclamation Operations Permits and Coal Exploration Systems Under Regulatory Programs,
        30 C.F.R. Part 795—Small Operator Assistance (July 1, 1980 ed.) (OSM)
    (a.) 30 C.F.R. § 795.1 through § 795.4
    (b.) § 795.16 Data requirements
    (c.) § 795.17 Qualified laboratories
    (d.) § 795.18 and § 795.19
(5.) Subchapter K, Permanent Program Performance Standards, Surface Mining Activities, Part 816.
    (a.) Hydrologic balance: Water quality standards and effluent limitations.
        30 C.F.R. § 816.42 (July 1, 1980 ed.) (OSM).
    (b.) Hydrologic balance: Surface and ground water monitoring
        30 C.F.R. § 816.52 (July 1, 1980 ed.) (OSM)
(6.) Subchapter K, Permanent Program Performance Standards, Underground Mining Activities, Part 817.
    (a.) Hydrologic balance: Water Quality standards and effluent limitations.
        30 C.F.R. § 817.42 (July 1, 1980 ed.) (OSM)
    (b.) Hydrologic balance: Surface and ground water monitoring.
        30 C.F.R. § 817.52 (July 1, 1980 ed., as amended on November 20, 1980, 45 Fed. Reg. 76932, 76935)
(7.) Surface Mining and Reclamation Operations; Interim and Permanent Regulatory Program; Notice of Suspension and Withdrawal of Certain Rules in 30 C.F.R. Chapter VII.
        44 Fed. Reg. 77440, 77451–55 (December 31, 1979), as corrected by 45 Fed. Reg. 6913 (January 30, 1980), and 45 Fed. Reg. 51547, 51549 (August 4, 1980) (OSM).
    (a.) Suspension of 30 C.F.R. § 715.17(a)(1) and 30 C.F.R. § 717.17(a)(3)(i) (44 Fed. Reg. 77451–52 and 45 Fed Reg. 6913)
    (b.) Suspension of 30 C.F.R. § 816.42(b) and 30 C.F.R. § 817.42(a)(1) and (7) (45 Fed. Reg. 6913 and 51547, 51549)
E. *Safe Drinking Water Regulations*
    (1.) National Interim Primary Drinking Water Regulations.
        40 C.F.R. Part 141 (July 1, 1980 ed., as amended on August 27, 1980, 45 Fed. Reg. 57332 *et seq.*) (Environmental Protection Agency) including:
    (a.) Subpart C—Monitoring and Analytical Requirements.
        40 C.F.R. § 141.21 *et seq.*
    (b.) Subpart E—Special Monitoring Regulations for Organic Chemicals.
        40 C.F.R. § 141.40 *et seq.*
    (2.) National Secondary Drinking Water Regulations.
        40 C.F.R. Part 143 (July 1, 1980 ed.) (Environmental Protection Agency)
F. *Bottled Drinking Water Regulations*
    (1.) Quality Standards for Foods With No Identity Standards, Part 103, Subpart B—Standards of Quality.
        21 C.F.R. § 103.35 (April 1, 1980 ed.) (Department of Health and Human Services, Food and Drug Administration)
    (2.) Processing and Bottling of Bottled Drinking Water.
        40 C.F.R. Part 129 (April 1, 1980 ed.) (Department of Health and Human Services, Food and Drug Administration)

TABLE E.   FEDERAL REGULATIONS REFERRING TO WATER METHODS—*Continued*

G. *Ocean Dumping Permit Program Regulations*
  (1.) Criteria for the Evaluation of Permit Applications for Ocean Dumping of Materials.
      40 C.F.R. Part 227 (July 1, 1980 ed.) (Environmental Protection Agency)
  (2.) Criteria for the Management of Disposal Sites for Ocean Dumping.
      40 C.F.R. Part 228 (July 1, 1980 ed. List of dumping sites at § 228.12 was amended on
      December 9, 1980 (45 Fed. Reg. 81042, 81044) (Environmental Protection Agency)

---

[1] The complete text of Table I., which represents the basic reference source of Federal regulations approving and citing water methods, is presented in this Supplement at page S4.

METHODS

I. METALS

NOTE: The distinction between dissolved and total metal concentration is that for dissolved metal the sample is filtered through a 0.45 micrometer filter *before* acidification.

Palladium
(Atomic Absorption, Direct Aspiration)*

Optimum Concentration Range: 0.5–15 mg/l using a wavelength of 247.6 nm

Sensitivity: 0.25 mg/l

Detection Limit: 0.1 mg/l

Preparation of Standard Solution

1. Stock Solution: Dissolve 0.1000 g of palladium wire in a minimum volume of aqua regia and evaporate just to dryness. Add 5 ml conc. HCl and 25 ml deionized water and warm until dissolution is complete. Dilute to 100 ml with deionized water (1 ml = 1 mg Pd).

2. A standard AAS solution of palladous chloride, $PdCl_2$, 1000 mg/l in aqueous matrix is available from Alfa Products, Beverly, Massachusetts 01915. Cat. #88085.

3. Prepare dilutions of the stock solution to be used as calibration standards at the time of analysis. The calibration standards should be prepared to contain 0.5% (v/v) HNO_3.

Sample Preservation

1. For sample handling and preservation, see part 4.1 of the Atomic Absorption Methods section of the EPA manual* †.

Sample Preparation

1. Transfer a representative aliquot of the well mixed sample to a Griffin beaker and add 3 ml of conc. distilled HNO_3. Place the beaker on a steam bath and evaporate to near dryness. Cool the beaker and cautiously add a 5 ml portion of aqua regia. (See below for preparation of aqua regia.‡) Cover the beaker with a watch glass and return to the steam bath. Continue heating the covered beaker for 30 minutes. Remove cover and evaporate to near dryness. Cool and add 1:1 redistilled HNO_3 (1 ml per 100 ml dilution). Wash down the beaker walls and watch glass with distilled water and filter the sample to remove silicates and other insoluble material that could clog the atomizer. Adjust the volume to some predetermined value based on the expected metal concentration. The sample is now ready for analysis.

Instrumental Parameters (General)

1. Palladium hollow cathode lamp
2. Wavelength: 247.6 nm
3. Fuel: Acetylene
4. Oxidant: Air
5. Type of flame: Oxidizing

---

* "Methods for Chemical Analysis of Water and Wastes, March 1979," U.S. Environmental Protection Agency, Environmental Monitoring and Support Laboratory (EMSL), (EPA-600/4-79-020).

† Essentially equivalent procedures are given in Sections 301 and 302, pp. 141ff, *Standard Methods*, 15th edition.

‡ Aqua regia—Prepare immediately before use by carefully adding three volumes of conc. HCl to one volume of conc. HNO_3.

Analysis Procedure

1. For analysis procedure and calculation, see "Direct Aspiration," part 9.1 of the Atomic Absorption Methods section of the EPA manual* §.

---

§ This procedure is essentially equivalent to that given in Section 303A.3, p. 154, *Standard Methods*, 15th edition.

Note

1. For concentrations of palladium below 0.25 mg/l, the furnace procedure, below, is recommended.

Precision and Accuracy

1. Precision and accuracy data are not available at this time.

Palladium
(Atomic Absorption, Furnace Technique)*

Optimum Concentration Range: 20–400 µg/l

Detection Limit: 5 µg/l

Preparation of Standard Solution

1. Stock solution: Prepare as described under "direct aspiration method."
2. Prepare dilutions of the stock solution to be used as calibration standards at the time of analysis. These solutions are also to be used for "standard additions."
3. The calibration standard should be diluted to contain 0.5% (v/v) HNO_3.

Sample Preservation

1. For sample handling and preservation, see part 4.1 of the Atomic Absorption Methods section of the EPA manual* †.

Sample Preparation

1. Prepare as described under "direct aspiration method." Sample solution for analysis should contain 0.5% (v/v) HNO_3.

---

* "Methods for Chemical Analysis of Water and Wastes, March 1979," U.S. Environmental Protection Agency, Environmental Monitoring and Support Laboratory (EMSL), (EPA-600/4-79-020).

† Essentially equivalent procedures are given in Sections 301 and 302, pp. 141ff, *Standard Methods*, 15th edition.

Instrument Parameters (General)

1. Drying Time and Temp: 30 sec–125° C.
2. Ashing Time and Temp: 30 sec–1000° C.
3. Atomizing Time and Temp: 10 sec–2800° C.
4. Purge Gas Atmosphere: Argon
5. Wavelength: 247.6 nm
6. Other operating parameters should be set as specified by the particular instrument manufacturer.

Analysis Procedure

1. For the analysis procedure and the calculation, see "Furnace Procedure" part 9.3 of the Atomic Absorption Methods section of the EPA manual* ‡.

Notes

1. The above concentration values and instrument conditions are for a Perkin-Elmer HGA-2100, based on the use of 20 µl injection, continuous flow purge gas and pyrolytic graphite. Smaller size furnace devices or those employing faster rates of atomization can be operated using lower atomization temperatures for shorter time periods than the above recommended settings.

---

‡ Reproduced below.

2. The use of background correction is recommended.

3. Nitrogen may also be used as the purge gas.

4. For every sample matrix analyzed, verification is necessary to determine that method of standard addition is not required (see part 5.2.1 of the Atomic Absorption Methods section of the EPA manual* ‡).

5. If method of standard addition is required, follow the procedure given in part 8.5 of the Atomic Absorption Methods section of the EPA manual* ‡.

Precision and Accuracy

1. Precision and accuracy data are not available at this time.

---

* "Methods for Chemical Analysis of Water and Wastes, March 1979," U.S. Environmental Protection Agency, Environmental Monitoring and Support Laboratory (EMSL), (EPA-600/4-79-020).

‡ Reproduced below.

9.3 Furnace Procedure: Furnace devices (flameless atomization) are a most useful means of extending detection limits. Because of differences between various makes and models of satisfactory instruments, no detailed operating instructions can be given for each instrument. Instead, the analyst should follow the instructions provided by the manufacturer of his particular instrument and use as a guide the temperature settings and other instrument conditions listed on the individual analysis sheets which are recommended for the Perkin-Elmer HGA-2100. In addition, the following points may be helpful.

9.3.1 With flameless atomization, background correction becomes of high importance especially below 350 nm. This is because certain samples, when atomized, may absorb or scatter light from the hollow cathode lamp. It can be caused by the presence of gaseous molecular species, salt particules, or smoke in the sample beam. If no correction is made, sample absorbance will be greater than it should be, and the analytical result will be erroneously high.

9.3.2 If during atomization all the analyte is not volatilized and removed from the furnace, memory effects will occur. This condition is dependent on several factors such as the volatility of the element and its chemical form, whether pyrolytic graphite is used, the rate of atomization and furnace design. If this situation is detected through blank burns, the tube should be cleaned by operating the furnace at full power for the required time period as needed at regular intervals in the analytical scheme.

9.3.3 Some of the smaller size furnace devices, or newer furnaces equipped with feedback temperature control (Instrumentation Laboratories MODEL 555, Perkin-Elmer MODELS HGA 2200 and HGA 76B, and Varian MODEL CRA-90) employing faster rates of atomization, can be operated using lower atomization temperatures for shorter time periods than those listed in this manual.

9.3.4 Although prior digestion of the sample in many cases is not required providing a representative aliquot of sample can be pipeted into the furnace, it will provide for a more uniform matrix and possibly lessen matrix effects.

9.3.5 Inject a measured microliter aliquot of sample into the furnace and atomize. If the concentration found is greater than the highest standard, the sample should be diluted in the same acid matrix and reanalyzed. The use of multiple injections can improve accuracy and help detect furnace pipetting errors.

9.3.6 To verify the absence of interference, follow the procedure as given in part 5.2.1.

9.3.7 A check standard should be run approximately after every 10 sample injections. Standards are run in part to monitor the life and performance of the graphite tube. Lack of reproducibility or significant change in the signal for the standard indicates that the tube should be replaced. Even though tube life depends on sample matrix and atomization temperature, a conservative estimate would be that a tube will last at least 50 firings. A pyrolytic-coating would extend that estimate by a factor of 3.

9.3.8 Calculation—For determination of metal concentration by the furnace: Read the metal value in μg/l from the calibration curve or directly from the readout system of the instrument.

9.3.8.1 If different size furnace injection volumes are used for samples than for standards:

$$\mu\text{g/l of metal in sample} = Z\left(\frac{S}{U}\right)$$

where:

$Z = \mu$g/l of metal read from calibration curve or readout system
$S = $ ul volume standard injected into furnace for calibration curve
$U = $ ul volume of sample injected for analysis

9.3.8.2 If dilution of sample was required but sample injection volume same as for standard:

$$\mu\text{g/l of metal sample} = Z\left(\frac{C + B}{C}\right)$$

where:

$Z = \mu$g/l metal in diluted aliquot from calibration curve

$B = $ ml of deionized distilled water used for dilution
$C = $ ml of sample aliquot

9.3.9 For sample containing particulates:

$$\mu\text{g/l of metal in sample} = Z\left(\frac{V}{C}\right)$$

where:

$Z = \mu$g/l of metal in processed sample from calibration curve (See 9.3.8.1)
$V = $ final volume of processed sample in ml
$C = $ ml of sample aliquot processed

9.3.10 For solid samples: Report all concentrations as mg/kg dry weight.

9.3.10.1 Dry sample:

$$\text{mg metal/kg sample} = \frac{\left(\dfrac{Z}{1,000}\right)V}{D}$$

where:

$Z = \mu$g/l of metal in processed sample from calibration curve (See 9.3.8.1)
$V = $ final volume of processed sample in ml
$D = $ weight of dry sample in grams

9.3.10.2 Wet sample:

$$\text{mg metal/kg sample} = \frac{\left(\dfrac{Z}{1,000}\right)V}{W \times P}$$

where:

$Z = \mu$g/l of metal in processed sample from calibration curve (See 9.3.8.1)
$V = $ final volume of processed sample in ml
$W = $ weight of wet sample in grams
$P = \%$ solids

5.2 Flameless Atomization

5.2.1 Although the problem of oxide formation is greatly reduced with furnace procedures because atomization occurs in an inert atmosphere, the technique is still subject to chemical and matrix interferences. The composition of the sample matrix can have a major effect on the analysis. It is those effects which must be determined and taken into consideration in the analysis of each different matrix encountered. To help verify the absence of matrix or chemical interference use the following procedure. Withdraw from the sample two equal aliquots. To one of the aliquots add a known amount of analyte and dilute both aliquots to the same predetermined volume. [The dilution volume should be based on the analysis of the undiluted sample. Preferably, the dilution should be 1:4 while keeping in mind the optimum concentration range of the analysis. Under no circumstances should the dilution be less than 1:1]. The diluted aliquots should then be analyzed and the unspiked results multiplied by the dilution factor should be compared to the original determination. Agreement of the results (within ±10%) indicates the absence of interference. Comparison of the actual signal from the spike to the expected response from the analyte in an aqueous standard should help confirm the finding from the dilution analysis. Those samples which indicate the presence of interference, should be tested in one or more of the following ways.

a. The samples should be successively diluted and reanalyzed to determine if the interference can be eliminated.

b. The matrix of the sample should be modified in the furnace. Examples are the addition of ammonium nitrate to remove alkali chlorides, ammonium phosphate to retain cadmium, and nickel nitrate for arsenic and selenium analyses [ATOMIC ABSORPTION NEWSLETTER Vol. 14, No. 5, p 127, Sept-Oct 1975]. The mixing of hydrogen with the inert purge gas has also been used to suppress chemical interference. The hydrogen acts as a reducing agent and aids in molecular dissociation.

c. Analyze the sample by method of standard additions while noting the precautions and limitations of its use (See 8.5).

8.5 Method of Standard Additions: In this method, equal volumes of sample are added to a deionized distilled water blank and to three standards containing different known amounts of the test element. The volume of the blank and the standards must be the same. The absorbance of each solution is determined and then plotted on the vertical axis of a graph, with the concentrations of the known standards plotted on the horizontal axis. When the resulting line is extrapolated back to zero absorbance, the point of interception of the abscissa is the concentration of the unknown. The abscissa on the left of the ordinate is scaled the same as on the right side, but in the opposite direction from the ordinate. An example of a plot so obtained is shown in Fig. 1. The method of standard additions can be very useful, however, for the results to be valid the following limitations must be taken into consideration:

a) the absorbance plot of sample and standards must be linear over the concentration range of concern. For best results the slope of the plot should be nearly the same as the slope of the aqueous standard curve.

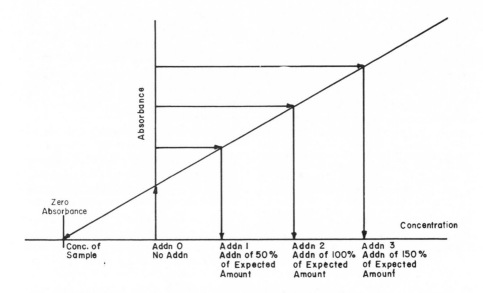

Figure 1. Standard addition plot.

If the slope is significantly different (more than 20%) caution should be exercised.

b) the effect of the interference should not vary as the ratio of analyte concentration to sample matrix changes and the standard addition should respond in a similar manner as the analyte.

c) the determination must be free of spectral interference and corrected for nonspecific background interference.

Uranium in Drinking Water—Radiochemical Method*

1. Scope and Application

1.1 This method covers the measurement of total uranium alpha particle activity in drinking water. Most drinking water sources, especially ground water sources, contain soluble carbonates and bicarbonates which complex and keep uranium in the water in solution.

1.2 Uranium isotopic abundances in drinking water sources are apt to be present in ratios different from the ratios in the deposits from which the uranium entered the water sources. The two predominant natural alpha emitting isotopes of uranium are uranium-234 and uranium-238. Uranium-238 is the predominant mass abundant isotope; greater than 99% compared to about 0.006% for uranium-234. However, uranium-234 has a specific activity for alpha particle emission that is 1.8×10^4 times greater than that of

*"Prescribed Procedures for Measurement of Radioactivity in Drinking Water." Environmental Monitoring and Support Laboratory, Environmental Protection Agency, EPA-600/4-80-032, August 1980.

uranium-238. For an equilibrium condition, the activity of the uranium-234 is equal to that of the uranium-238. Therefore, the uranium mass concentration in water is not related to the alpha particle activity of the water.

1.3 The Drinking Water Regulations under the Safe Drinking Water Act, PL 93-523, require a measurement of uranium for drinking water samples that have a gross alpha activity greater than 15 pCi/l. A mass uranium concentration measurement of a water sample cannot be converted to uranium alpha activity without first analyzing for isotopic abundances. Therefore, a method such as this one is needed to determine the total uranium alpha activity of the sample, without doing an isotopic uranium analysis.

2. Summary of Method

2.1 The water sample is made acid by adding HCl and the sample is boiled to eliminate carbonate and bicarbonate ions. Uranium is coprecipitated with ferric hydroxide and separated from the sample. The uranium is then separated from other radionuclides which were carried down with the ferric hydroxide by dissolving the hydroxide precipitate in $8N$ HCl, putting the solution through an anion exchange column, washing the column with $8N$ HCl, and finally eluting the uranium with $0.1N$ HCl. The uranium eluate is evaporated and the uranium chemical form is converted to nitrate. The residue is transferred to a stainless steel planchet, dried, flamed, and counted for alpha particle activity.

2.2 Uranium recovery is determined with blank samples spiked with known amounts of uranium and taken through the procedure as a regular sample.

2.3 Counting efficiency is determined by transferring measured aliquots of an uranium standard to a planchet, diluting

with 6–8 ml of a 1 mg/ml HIO_3 solution in $4N$ HNO_3, evaporating to dryness, flaming the planchet, and counting in an alpha counter.

3. Sample Handling and Preservation

3.1 Although carbonate ions in a water sample will help to keep uranium in solution, the addition of extra carbonate or bicarbonate ions to the sample as a preservative is not recommended because an increased carbonate concentration in the sample may cause some precipitation. Therefore, it is recommended that samples be preserved with HCl to pH 2 at the time of collection.

3.2 A sample size of at least 1 liter should be collected for uranium analysis.

4. Interferences

4.1 The only alpha-emitting radionuclide that may come through the chemistry and cause interference would be protactinium-231. However, protactinium-231 results from the decay of uranium-235, a low abundance natural isotope of uranium, and would therefore cause only a very small interference.

4.2 Since uranium is a naturally occurring radionuclide, reagents must be checked for uranium contamination by analyzing a complete reagent blank by the same procedure as used for the samples.

5. Apparatus—See Appendix D* † for details and specifications

5.1 Gas-flow proportional counting system or

5.2 Scintillation detection system

---

* "Prescribed Procedures for Measurement of Radioactivity in Drinking Water." Environmental Monitoring and Support Laboratory, Environmental Protection Agency, EPA-600/4-80-032, August 1980.

† Reproduced on p. S40.

5.3 Glassware

5.4 Electric hot plate

5.5 Ion exchange column: approximately 13 mm (i.d.) × 150 mm long with a 100 ml reservoir.

5.6 Stainless steel counting planchets, 2 inch diameter by ¼ inch deep.

5.7 Millipore filter apparatus, 47 mm.

6. Reagents

6.1 All chemicals should be of reagent grade or equivalent whenever they are commercially available.

6.2 Ammonium hydroxide, $6N$: Mix 2 volumes $15N$ NH_4OH (conc.) with 3 volumes of water (carbonate-free.)

6.3 Anion exchange resin—Strongly basic, styrene, quaternary ammonium salt, 4% crosslinked, 100–200 mesh, chloride form (such as Dowex 1 × 4, or equivalent).

6.4 Ferric chloride carrier, 20 mg Fe^{+3}/ml: Dissolve 9.6g of $FeCl_3 \cdot 6H_2O$ in 100 ml of $0.5\ N$ HCl.

6.5 Hydriodic acid: HI (conc.), sp. gr. 1.5, 47%.

6.6 Hydrochloric acid, $12N$: HCl (conc.), sp. gr. 1.19, 37.2%.

6.7 Hydrochloric acid, $8N$: Mix 2 volumes $12N$ HCl (conc.) with 1 volume of water.

6.8 Hydrochloric acid, $6N$: Mix 1 volume $12N$ HCl (conc.) with 1 volume of water.

6.9 Hydrochloric acid, $0.1N$:—Mix 1 volume $0.5N$ HCl with 4 volumes of water.

6.10 Iodic acid, 1 mg/ml: Dissolve 100 mg HIO_3 in 100 ml $4N$ HNO_3.

6.11 Nitric acid, $16N$: HNO_3 (conc.), sp. gr. 1.42, 70.4%.

6.12 Nitric acid, $4N$: Mix 1 volume $16N$ HNO_3 (conc.) with 3 volumes of water.

6.13 Sodium hydrogen sulfite, $NaHSO_3$.

6.14 Sodium hydrogen sulfite, 1% in

HCl: Dissolve 1g $NaHSO_3$ in 100 ml $6N$ HCl.

7. Calibrations

7.1 Determine a counting efficiency (E), for a known amount of standard uranium (about 1000 dpm) evaporated from a 6–8 ml volume of a 1 mg/ml HIO_3 solution in a 2 inch diameter stainless steel planchet. If the standard solution is an HCl solution, then aliquot portions of that solution must be converted to nitrate/HNO_3 solutions, eliminating all chloride ions from the solutions. This can be done by three successive evaporations after adding 5 ml portions of $16N$ HNO_3 to aliquot portions of the standard in small beakers (avoiding dry baking of the evaporated residue). The final solutions of the standard aliquots are made by adding 2 ml $4N$ HNO_3 solution to the third evaporated residues. Transfer the uranium standard aliquot solutions to 2 inch diameter stainless steel planchets.

Complete the transfer by rinsing the beakers two times with 2 ml portions of $4N$ HNO_3 and evaporate to dryness. Flame the planchets and count for at least 50 minutes for alpha particle activity. A reagent blank should be run along with the standard aliquots and should be alpha counted.

$$\text{Efficiency, cpm/dpm, (E)} = \frac{A - B}{C}$$

where:

A = gross cpm for standard
B = cpm for instrument background
C = dpm of standard use

7.2 A uranium recovery factor, R, is determined by the following procedure: Spike one liter tap water samples with aliquots of uranium standard solution (500–1000 dpm per sample). Take these spiked samples and a tap water blank through the entire procedure and count the separated and evaporated uranium for alpha particle activity.

$$\text{Recovery factor, (R)} = \frac{(F - B)}{CE}$$

where:

C = dpm of uranium standard added
F = gross cpm of spiked sample
B = cpm of reagent blank
E = efficiency factor, cpm/dpm

8. Procedure

8.1 Measure the volume of approximately one liter of the water sample to be analyzed.

8.1.2 If the sample has not been acidified, add 5 ml 12N HCl and 1 ml ferric chloride carrier.

8.1.3 Mix the sample completely and use pH paper to check the hydrogen-ion concentration. If the pH is > 1, add 12N HCl until it reaches this value.

8.1.4 Cover with a watch glass and heat the water sample to boiling for 20 minutes.

8.1.5 The pH must be checked again after boiling and if it is > 1, 12N HCl must be added to bring the pH back to 1.

8.1.6 While the sample is still boiling gently add 6N NH$_4$OH to the sample from a polyethylene squeeze bottle with the bottle delivery tube inserted between the watch glass and the pouring lip of the beaker. The boiling action of the sample provides sufficient stirring action. Add 6N NH$_4$OH until turbidity persists while boiling continues; then add an additional 10 ml (estimated addition from the squeeze bottle).

8.1.7 Continue to boil the sample for 10 minutes more; then set it aside for 30 minutes to cool and settle.

8.1.8 After the sample has settled sufficiently, decant and filter the supernate through a 47 mm 0.45 micron membrane filter, using the larger millipore filtering apparatus.

8.1.9 Slurry the remaining precipitate, transfer to the filtering apparatus and filter with suction.

8.1.10 Place the filtering apparatus over a clean 250 ml filtering flask, add 25 ml 8N HCl to dissolve precipitate, and filter the solution.

8.1.11 Add another 25 ml 8N HCl to wash the filter, and then filter.

8.1.12 Transfer solution to the 100 ml reservoir of the ion exchange column.

8.1.13 Rinse the side arm filtering flask twice with 25 ml portions of 8N HCl. Combine in the ion exchange reservoir.

8.2 Anion Exchange Separation

8.2.1 Prepare the column by slurrying the anion exchange resin with 8N HCl and pouring it onto a column of about 13 mm inside diameter. The height of the resin bed should be about 80 mm.

8.2.2 Pass the sample solution through the anion exchange resin column at a flow rate not to exceed 5 ml/min.

8.2.3 After the sample has passed through the column, elute the iron (and plutonium if present) with 6 column volumes of 8N HCl containing 1 ml 47% HI per 9 ml of 8N HCl (freshly prepared).

8.2.4 Wash the column with an additional two column volumes of 8N HCl.

8.2.5 Elute the uranium with six column volumes of 0.1N HCl.

8.2.6 Evaporate the acid eluate to near dryness and convert the residue salts to nitrates by three successive treatments with 5 ml portions of 16N HNO$_3$, evaporating to near dryness each time.

8.2.7 Dissolve the residue (may be very little visible residue) in 2 ml 4N HNO$_3$.

8.2.8 Transfer the residue solution, using a Pasteur pipet, to a marked planchet, and complete the transfer by rinsing the sample beaker three times with 2 ml portions of 4N HNO$_3$.

8.2.9 Evaporate the contents in the planchet to dryness, flame to remove traces of HIO$_3$, cool, and count for alpha particle activity.

8.3 Column Regeneration

8.3.1 Pass three column volumes of 1% NaHSO$_3$ in 6N HCl through the column.

8.3.2 Pass six column volumes of 6N HCl through the column.

8.3.3 Pass three column volumes of water through the column.

8.3.4 Pass six column volumes of 8N HCl through the column to equilibrate and ready the resin for the next set of samples.

9. Calculations

Uranium alpha activity, pCi/l

$$= \frac{(S - B) \times 1000}{2.22 \times E\ R\ V}$$

where:

S = gross cpm for sample
B = cpm of reagent blank
V = volume of sample used, ml
E = efficiency, cpm/dpm
R = recovery factor
2.22 = conversion factor for dpm/pCi

10. Precision and Accuracy

In a single laboratory test of this method, a stock uranium solution was prepared using tap water and spiked with an NBS uranium standard. The calculated concentration was 26.7 pCi/l. This stock solution was acidified with HCl as a preservative. Nine 1-liter aliquots were withdrawn and the procedure tested. Individual results were 22.4, 22.5, 24.0, 25.9, 26.9, 26.5, 24.6, 25.7 and 23.9 pCi/l. The average concentration was 24.7 pCi/l with a standard deviation of 1.7 pCi/l. From these data, the method shows a negative 7.4% bias and a precision of ±6.7% without the correction of the recovery factor.

References

1. Bishop, C. T., et. al. "Radiometric Method for the Determination of Uranium in Water", EPA 600/7-79-093, EMSL-LV, April 1979.
2. Edwards, K. W. "Isotopic Analysis of Uranium in Natural Waters by Alpha Spectrometry," Radiochemical Analysis of Water, Geological Survey Water—Supply Paper 1696-F, U.S. Government Printing Office, Washington, D.C., 1968.

Uranium in Drinking Water—Fluorometric Method*

1. Scope and Application

1.1 The method covers the determination of soluble uranium in waters at concentrations greater than 0.1 μg/l. There is no upper limit, since waters whose uranium concentrations exceed the upper limit of the measurement range need only be diluted to be within this range.

1.2 Uranium is present in surface and ground waters at concentrations generally less than 20 μg/l. This method is applicable for the monitoring of water discharges from industries related to the uranium fuel

---

* "Prescribed Procedures for Measurement of Radioactivity in Drinking Water." Environmental Monitoring and Support Laboratory, Environmental Protection Agency, EPA-600/4-80-032, August 1980.

cycle. Since the method measures the mass of uranium, it is applicable to the assessment of chemical toxicity. The method can be indirectly used for the assessment of radiation effects if the isotopic composition is known or measured.

2. Summary of Method

Uranium is concentrated by coprecipitation with aluminum phosphate. The aluminum phosphate is dissolved in dilute nitric acid containing magnesium nitrate as a salting agent and the coprecipitated uranium is extracted into ethyl acetate. After the ethyl acetate is removed by evaporation, the extracted residue is dissolved in nitric acid and diluted to volume in a small volumetric flask. Aliquots are transferred to each of two fusion dishes and dried. To one dish is added a known mass of uranium (0.1 µg) and dried. Flux containing sodium fluoride is added to each of the dishes, fused at a prescribed temperature, cooled and read in a fluorometer. The use of the standard addition technique corrects for any interference that may coextract with uranium.

3. Interferences

3.1 The fluorescence of uranium in a fluoride matrix can be quenched or enhanced by either cations or anions. When uranium is present in low concentration (less than 20 µg/l) these interferences can be eliminated by the coprecipitation of uranium on aluminum phosphate and subsequent uranium extraction into ethyl acetate.

3.2 Carbonate ions form soluble uranium complexes which prevent the coprecipitation on aluminum phosphate. Carbonates are removed by acidification and expelled from solution as volatile carbon dioxide.

4. Apparatus

See Appendix D* † for details and specifications.

4.1 Fluorometer, Jarrell-Ash or equivalent.

4.2 Dish forming die, Cat. No. 26100, Fisher Scientific.

4.3 Fusion dish blanks—Gold or Platinum 0.015 in. thickness × 0.75 in. diameter.

4.4 Muffle furnace—controlled temperature.

4.5 Microliter pipette—100 µl.

4.6 Glassware.

5. Reagents

5.1 Purity of Reagents—Reagent grade chemicals shall be used in all tests. Unless otherwise indicated, it is intended that all reagents shall conform to the specifications of the committee on analytical reagents of the American Chemical Society. Other grades may be used provided it is first ascertained that the reagent is of sufficiently high purity to permit its use without lessening the accuracy of the determination.

5.2 Purity of Water. Unless otherwise indicated, reference to water shall be understood to mean conforming to ASTM Specification D 1193, Type III.

5.3 Aluminum nitrate, 0.08M: Dissolve 15 g $Al(NO_3)_3 \cdot 9H_2O$ in 500 ml of water.

5.4 Ammonium hydroxide, 15N: NH_4OH (conc.) sp.gr. 0.90, 56.6%.

5.5 Diammonium hydrogen phosphate 0.11M: Dissolve 7.26 g $(NH_4)_2HPO_4$ in 500 ml water.

5.6 Ethyl acetate, $CH_3COOC_2H_5$, reagent grade.

---

* "Prescribed Procedures for Measurement of Radioactivity in Drinking Water." Environmental Monitoring and Support Laboratory, Environmental Protection Agency, EPA-600/4-80-032, August 1980.

† Reproduced on p. S40.

5.7 Flux: Mix together 9 parts NaF, 45.5 parts Na_2CO_3, 45.5 parts K_2CO_3 by weight in a ball mill.

5.8 Magnesium nitrate, $3.5M$: Dissolve 449 g $Mg(NO_3)_2 \cdot 6H_2O$ in 350 ml water containing 32 ml $16N$ HNO_3. Warm if necessary to dissolve. Cool and dilute to 500 ml.

5.9 Nitric acid, $16N$: HNO_3 (conc.), sp. gr. 1.42, 70.4%.

5.10 Nitric acid, $0.1N$: Mix 1 volume $16N$ HNO_3 (conc.) with 159 volumes of water.

5.11 Phenolphthalein (5 g/l): Dissolve 0.5 g phenolphthalein in 50 ml ethanol (95%) and dilute to 100 ml with water.

5.12 Sodium thiosulfate, $Na_2S_2O_3$: crystal.

5.13 Uranium standard stock solution. 100 μg/ml. Weigh out 0.1179 g U_3O_8 into a 100 ml beaker and dissolve in 10 ml $1N$ HNO_3, warming on a hot plate as required. Transfer to a 100 ml volumetric flask with water and dilute to volume.

5.14 Uranium standard solution, 10 μg/l. Transfer 5.0 ml of the 1000 μg/l uranium solution to a 500 ml volumetric flask and dilute to volume with $0.1N$ HNO_3.

5.15 Uranium standard solution, 1 μg/l. Transfer 10.0 ml of the 10 μg/l uranium solution to a 100 ml volumetric flask and dilute to volume with $0.1N$ HNO_3.

5.16 Uranium standard solution, 0.1 μg/l: Transfer 10.0 ml of the 1.0 μg/l uranium solution to a 100 ml volumetric flask and dilute to volume with $0.1N$ HNO_3.

6. Procedure

6.1 Direct Analysis (Samples greater than 20 μg/l).

6.1.1 Transfer two 100 μl aliquots of the filtered sample to each of two gold dishes and evaporate to dryness under heat lamps.

6.1.2 To one of the gold dishes add 100 μl of a uranium standard (0.1 μg/ml for

samples 20–400 μg/l or 1.0 μg/ml for samples greater than 400 μg/l).

6.1.3 Evaporate to dryness under a heat lamp.

6.1.4 Using a balance sensitive to at least one milligram, weigh out 400 ± 4 mg flux into each of the two gold dishes.

6.1.5 Prepare a blank flux sample by weighing out 400 ± 4 mg flux into a clean gold dish.

6.1.6 Place the three gold dishes into a stainless steel support and place in a preheated muffle furnace at 625° C for 15 minutes.

6.1.7 Remove from furnace and cool in a desiccator for 30 minutes.

6.1.8 Read in a fluorometer as directed in Section 7.0.

6.2 Coprecipitation (Samples less than 20 μg/l).

6.2.1 Measure a 1 liter aliquot of filtered water into a 1500 ml beaker.

6.2.2 Acidify with 2 ml $16N$ HNO_3 (This may be omitted if sample was previously acidified for preservation).

6.2.3 Add 5 ml each of the aluminum nitrate and diammonium hydrogen phosphate solutions and mix.

6.2.4 If sample was chlorinated as in the case of a drinking water sample, add one crystal of sodium thiosulfate and stir.

6.2.5 Heat to near boiling to expel dissolved carbon dioxide gas.

6.2.6 Add 5 drops of phenolphthalein indicator and neutralize to the pink end point using $15N$ NH_4OH.

6.2.7 Lower the heat and digest sample for 30 minutes.

6.2.8 Remove from heat, cool, and settle for one hour.

6.2.9 Decant and filter the clarified supernate through a 47 mm glass fiber filter, transferring the settled precipitate at the very end.

6.2.10 Wash beaker and filter with small portions of water.

6.2.11 Fold filter into thirds (similar to the folding of a letter) and transfer to a 50 ml screw cap centrifuge tube.

NOTE: If some of the precipitate remains on the inside edges of the filtering apparatus gently wipe with the folded filter before transferring to the centrifuge tube.

6.2.12 Add 15 ml 3.5M $Mg(NO_3)_2 \cdot 6H_2O$ to the centrifuge tube to dissolve the aluminum phosphate.

6.2.13 Add 10 ml ethyl acetate, securely cap the tube and mix thoroughly for one minute using a vortex mixer.

6.2.14 Centrifuge at 2000 rpm for 5 minutes.

6.2.15 Using a Pasteur transfer pipette, transfer about 9 ml of the top layer (ethyl acetate) to a 30 ml beaker.

6.2.16 Repeat steps 6.2.13 to 6.2.15 two more times.

6.2.17 Slowly evaporate the combined ethyl acetate fractions to dryness.

6.2.18 Add 1 ml 16N HNO_3 and dissolve residue.

6.2.19 Using the same Pasteur pipette, transfer the nitric acid to a 5 ml volumetric flask.

6.2.20 Add 1 ml of water to the beaker, wash down the sides of the beaker using the pipet, and transfer to the 5 ml volumetric flask.

6.2.21 Repeat 6.2.20 two more times.

6.2.22 Gently mix, cool, dilute to volume with water, and shake thoroughly.

6.2.23 Proceed with steps 6.1.1 through 6.1.8, using the 1.0 μg/ml uranium standard.

7. Fluorometric Determination

7.1 Place the gold dish containing the sample plus the uranium spike into the fluorometer.

7.2 Following the manufacturer's suggested technique, adjust the voltage to maximize the reading such as full scale deflection.

7.3 Remove the spiked sample, insert the background sample and adjust the null voltage to read zero.

7.4 Repeat steps 7.2 and 7.3 until no more voltage adjustments are required.

7.5 Insert the gold dish containing the sample only and record the output.

8. Calculations

8.1 The results of the analysis are expressed in micrograms per liter and are calculated as follows:

$$\text{Uranium, } \mu\text{g/l} = \frac{5\left[\dfrac{R_s - R_b}{R_{ss} - R_s}\right] \times a}{b \times V}$$

where:

R_s = Reading of the sample
R_b = Reading of the blank
R_{ss} = Reading of the spiked sample
a = Mass of the uranium spike, μg
b = Aliquot size of the concentrate, ml
V = Initial sample size in liters
5 = Volume of the volumetric flask, ml

8.2 In the case where the uranium concentration is greater than 20 μg/l and no concentration procedure is performed, the factors "5" and "b" of the above equation are deleted.

9. Precision and Accuracy

9.1 Precision

9.1.1 The single laboratory precision of the method was evaluated by replicate analyses of a spiked uranium sample at the 10 μg/l concentration. The standard deviation is calculated from the equation:

$$S = \left[\frac{\Sigma(X_i^2) - \dfrac{(\Sigma X_i)^2}{N}}{N - 1}\right]^{1/2}$$

where:

$\Sigma(X_i^2)$ = summation of the squares of the individual results

$(\Sigma X_i)^2$ = square of the summation of the individual results

N = number of results

9.1.2 The coefficient of variation (CV) is calculated from the equation.

$$CV = \frac{100\ S}{X}$$

where:

S = standard deviation from the above equation

X = mean value of the individual results

9.1.3 Using the above equations, the coefficient of variation has been estimated as ± 15%.

9.2 Accuracy or Bias

9.2.1 The single laboratory accuracy of the method was evaluated over the uranium concentration range of 1–10 $\mu g/l$. The percent accuracy was calculated from the equation:

$$\%\ \text{Accuracy} = \frac{100\ (X_i - X_t)}{X_t}$$

where:

X_i = determined value of individual sample

X_t = known value of the sample

9.2.2 The average percent accuracy, A, is calculated from the equation:

$$A = \frac{\Sigma\%\ \text{Accuracy}}{N}$$

where:

$\Sigma\%$ Accuracy = summation of the individual accuracy determinations

N = number of determinations

9.2.3 The single laboratory evaluation of the average percent accuracy is estimated to be ± 104%.

References

1. BARKER, F.B., et al., "Determination of Uranium in Natural Waters," Geol. Survey Water Supply Paper, 1696-C (1965).
2. BLANCHARD, R., "Uranium Decay Series Disequilibrium in Age Determination of Marine Calcium Carbonates," Ph.D. Thesis, Washington University, St. Louis, Mo. June 1963.
3. EDWARD, K.W., "Isotopic Analysis of Uranium in Natural Waters by Alpha Spectroscopy," Geological Survey Water Supply Paper 1696-F (1968).
4. GRIMALDI, F.S., et al., "Collected Papers on Methods of Analysis for Uranium and Thorium," Geological Survey Bulletin 1006 (1954).

APPENDIX D
LABORATORY APPARATUS SPECIFICATIONS

1. Gas-flow proportional counting system: A gas-flow proportional counting system may be used for the measurement of gross alpha and gross beta activities. The detector may be either a "windowless" (internal proportional counter) or a "thin window" type. A minimum shielding equivalent to 5 cm of lead should surround the detector. A cosmic (guard) detector operated in anticoincidence with the main sample detector will convert this system to a low-background beta counter (< 3 cpm). The system shall be such that the sensitivity of the radioanalysis of water

samples will meet or exceed the requirements of the drinking water promulgated standards. The instrument should have a lengthy voltage plateau for detecting alpha or beta radioactivity plus a scaler consisting of a register, power supply, and amplifier.

2. Scintillator detector system: For measurement of alpha activities a scintillation system designed for alpha counting may be substituted for the gas-flow proportional counter described. In such a system, a Mylar disc coated with a phosphor (silver-activated zinc sulfide) is placed directly on the sample or on the face of a photomultiplier tube, enclosed within a light-tight container, along with the appropriate electronics (high voltage supply, amplifier, timer, and scaler).

3. Gamma spectrometer systems: Either a sodium iodide (NaI(Tl)) crystal or a solid state lithium drifted germanium (Ge(Li)) detector used in conjunction with a multichannel analyzer is required if the laboratory is to be certified for analyses of photon emitters from man-made radionuclides.

If a sodium iodide detector is used, a 10 cm × 10 cm NaI cylindrical crystal is recommended, although, a 7.5 cm × 7.5 cm crystal is satisfactory. The detector must be shielded with a minimum of 10 cm of iron or equivalent. It is recommended that the distance from the center of the detector to any part of the shield should not be less than 30 cm. The multichannel analyzer, in addition to appropriate electronics, should contain a memory of not less than 200 channels.

A system with a lithium drifted germanium (Ge(Li)) detector may be used for measurement of these photon emitters if the efficiency of the detector is such that the sensitivity of the system meets the minimum detectable activity requirements.

4. Beta/Gamma coincidence scintillation system. Since iodine-131 has a distinctive beta-gamma decay chain and a high enough beta-particle energy to be efficiently detected, a beta/gamma coincidence technique can be employed for quantification. A system of high-resolution detectors and multichannel analyzers results in very low background.

5. Liquid scintillation spectrometer counting system. The measurement of low-energy beta emitters such as tritium or carbon-14 can be best determined by liquid scintillation counting. These instruments use an organic phosphor as the primary detector. This organic phosphor is combined with the sample in an appropriate solvent that achieves a uniform dispersion. The counting system normally uses two multiplier phototubes in coincidence, thus providing a lower background. In order to minimize detectable radioactivity, scintillation-grade organic phosphors and solvents, and low-potassium scintillation vials are used.

6. Scintillation cell system: For the specific measurement of radium-226 by the radon emanation method, a scintillation system designed to accept scintillation flasks ("Lucas cells") shall be used. The system consists of a light-tight enclosure capable of accepting the scintillation flasks, a detector (phototube), and the appropriate electronics (high voltage supply amplifier timers and scalers). The flasks (cells) required for this measurement may either be purchased from commercial suppliers or constructed according to published specifications.

7. Radon emanation apparatus: This specialized glassware apparatus consists of:

Radon bubbler — Figure 2.

Scintillation cell — Figure 3.

The glassware can be fabricated by

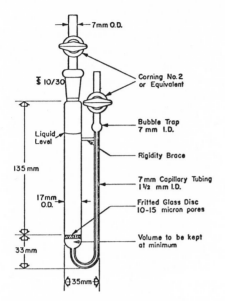

Figure 2. A typical radon bubbler.

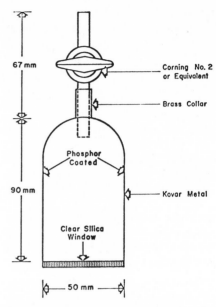

Figure 3. A typical scintillation cell for radon counting.

a competent glassblower, and the scintillation cell can be purchased from specified companies.

8. Fluorometer: An instrument to measure the fluorescence of a fused disc of a uranium compound exposed to ultraviolet light. The response to this excitation is proportional to the concentration of uranium in the drinking water sample. One of the specifications of the fluorometer is that it should be able to measure 0.0005 μg of uranium or less.

9. Analytical balance: Minimum scale readability, 0.1 mg.

10. Centrifuge:

10.1 General purpose table-top model with a maximum speed of at least 3,000 rpm and a loading option of 4 × 50 ml.

10.2 Floor model with a maximum speed of 2,000 rpm and a loading option of 4 × 250 ml centrifuge bottles.

11. pH meter: Accuracy, ±0.5 units. Scale readability, ±0.1 units. Instrument may be either line/bench or battery/portable.

12. Electric hot plate: This instrument should have a built-in stirrer, and stepless temperature controls which can be changed as heating requirements may demand.

13. Drying oven: The gravity convection type is recommended, having thermostatic controls to maintain desired temperature.

14. Mylar film: As a covering for precipitates to protect them during counting and storage, the thickness suggested is 0.0005 inches, in rolls of 1½ inch width.

15. Stainless steel counting planchets: These should be fabricated from uniform surface density stainless steel and capable of withstanding nitric acid and heat treatment. The planchets should be flat, have a

raised wall to contain the sample being evaporated and should be of the size determined by the inside diameter of the detector.

16. Drying lamps: As a minimum, these should consist of 250 watt infrared lamps with built-in reflectors that can be mounted on porcelain support stands.

17. Teflon filter holder: A fabricated device for filtering precipitates prior to mounting. These teflon units are to be made in dimensions compatible with the size of the plastic ring and disc mounts.

18. Plastic ring and disc mounts: These are plastic units molded of nylon in dimensions compatible with the size of the counting chamber of the counting instrument.

19. Desiccator:

Aluminum models, normally used for plastic ring and disc planchets.

Glass models, capable of holding a vacuum, and large enough to hold dried S.S. planchets until ready for counting.

20. Glassware: Borosilicate type glass. All glassware should meet Federal specifications. Beakers, 250 ml larger are required for specific analyses.

21. Glass fiber filters: These are type A-E, 47 mm in diameter.

22. Membrane filters: Metricel, 47 mm GA-6, 0.45 μ size.

23. Alpha sensitive phosphors—alpha phosphor disc, 24 mm ASP-4.

II. INORGANIC NON-METALS

Bromide
(Titrimetric)*

1. Scope and Application

1.1 This method is applicable to drinking, surface, and saline waters, domestic and industrial waste effluents.

1.2 The concentration range for this method is 2–20 mg bromide/l.

2. Summary of Method

2.1 After pretreatment to remove interferences, the sample is divided into two aliquots. One aliquot is analyzed for iodide by converting the iodide to iodate with bromine water and titrating iodometrically with phenylarsine oxide (PAO) or sodium thiosulfate. The other aliquot is analyzed for iodide plus bromide by converting these halides to iodate and bromate with calcium hypochlorite and titrating iodometrically with PAO or sodium thiosulfate. Bromide is then calculated by difference.

3. Sample Handling and Preservation

3.1 Store at 4°C and analyze as soon as possible.

4. Interferences

4.1 Iron, manganese and organic matter can interfere; however, the calcium oxide pretreatment removes or reduces these to insignificant concentrations.

4.2 Color interferes with the observation of indicator and bromine-water color changes. This interference is eliminated by

---

* "Methods for Chemical Analysis of Water and Wastes, 1974." U.S. Environmental Protection Agency, Environmental Monitoring and Support Laboratory (EMSL), (EPA-625/6-74-003a).

the use of a pH meter instead of a pH indicator and the use of standardized amounts of oxidant and oxidant-quencher.

5. Reagents

5.1 Acetic Acid Solution (1:8): Mix 100 ml of glacial acetic acid with 800 ml of distilled water.

5.2 Bromine Water: In a fume hood, add 0.2 ml bromine to 500 ml distilled water. Stir with a magnetic stirrer and a Teflon-coated stirring bar for several hours or until the bromine dissolves. Store in a glass-stoppered colored bottle.

5.3 Calcium Carbonate ($CaCO_3$): Powdered.

5.4 Calcium Hypochlorite Solution ($Ca(OCl)_2$): Add 35 g of $Ca(OCl)_2$ to approximately 800 ml of distilled water in a 1 liter volumetric flask. Stir on a magnetic stirrer for approximately 30 minutes. Dilute to 1 liter and filter. Store in a glass-stoppered, colored flask.

5.5 Calcium Oxide (CaO): Anhydrous, powdered.

5.6 Hydrochloric Acid Solution (1:4): Mix 100 ml of HCl (sp. gr. 1.19) with 400 ml of distilled water.

5.7 Potassium Iodide (KI): Crystals, ACS Reagent Grade.

5.8 Sodium Acetate Solution (275 g/l): Dissolve 275 g sodium acetate trihydrate ($NaC_2H_3O_2 \cdot 3H_2O$) in distilled water. Dilute to 1 liter and filter.

5.9 Sodium Chloride (NaCl): Crystals, ACS Reagent Grade.

5.10 Sodium Formate Solution (500 g/l): Dissolve 50 g sodium formate ($NaCHO_2$) in hot distilled water and dilute to 100 ml.

5.11 Sodium Molybdate Solution (10

g/l): Dissolve 1 g sodium molybdate ($Na_2MoO_4 \cdot 2H_2O$) in distilled water and dilute to 100 ml.

5.12 Sulfuric Acid Solution (1:4): Slowly add 200 ml H_2SO_4 (sp. gr. 1.84) to 800 ml of distilled water.

5.13 Phenylarsine Oxide (0.0375N): Hach Chemical Co., or equivalent. Standardize with 0.0375 N potassium biiodate (5.19, 5.23).

5.14 Phenylarsine Oxide Working Standard (0.0075 N): Transfer 100 ml of commercially available 0.0375 N phenylarsine oxide (5.13) to a 500 ml volumetric flask and dilute to the mark with distilled water. This solution should be prepared fresh daily.

5.15 Amylose Indicator: Mallinckrodt Chemical Works or equivalent.

5.16 Sodium Thiosulfate, Stock Solution, 0.75 N: Dissolve 186.14 g $Na_2S_2O_3 \cdot 5H_2O$ in boiled and cooled distilled water and dilute to 1 liter. Preserve by adding 5 ml chloroform.

5.17 Sodium Thiosulfate Standard Titrant, 0.0375 N: Prepare by diluting 50.0 ml of stock solution (5.16) to 1.0 liter. Preserve by adding 5 ml of chloroform. Standardize with 0.0375 N potassium biiodate (5.19, or 5.23).

5.18 Sodium Thiosulfate Working Standard (0.0075 N): Transfer 100 ml of sodium thiosulfate standard titrant (5.17) to a 500 ml volumetric flask and dilute to the mark with distilled water. This solution should be prepared fresh daily.

5.19 Potassium Biiodate Standard, 0.0375 N: Dissolve 4.873 g potassium biiodate, previously dried 2 hours at 103°C, in distilled water and dilute to 1.0 liter. Dilute 250 ml to 1.0 liter for 0.0375 N biiodate solution.

5.20 Starch Solution: Prepare an emulsion of 10 g of soluble starch in a mortar or beaker with a small quantity of distilled water. Pour this emulsion into 1 liter of boiling water, allow to boil a few minutes, and let settle overnight. Use the clear supernate. This solution may be preserved by the addition of 5 ml per liter of chloroform and storage in a 10°C refrigerator. Commercially available dry, powdered starch indicators may be used in place of starch solution.

5.21 Nitrogen Gas: Cylinder.

5.22 Potassium Fluoride ($KF \cdot 2H_2O$): ACS Reagent Grade.

5.23 Standardization of 0.0375 N Phenylarsine Oxide and 0.0375 N Sodium Thiosulfate: Dissolve approximately 2 g (± 1.0 g) KI (5.7) in 100 to 150 ml distilled water; add 10 ml H_2SO_4 solution (5.12) followed by 20 ml standard potassium biiodate solution (5.19). Place in dark for 5 minutes, dilute to 300 ml and titrate with the phenylarsine oxide (5.13) or sodium thiosulfate (5.17) to a pale straw color. Add a small scoop of indicator (5.15). Wait until homogeneous blue color develops and continue the titration drop by drop until the color disappears. Run in duplicate. Duplicate determinations should agree within ± 0.05 ml.

6. Procedure

6.1 Pretreatment

6.1.1 Add a visible excess of CaO (5.5) to 400 ml of sample. Stir or shake vigorously for approximately 5 minutes. Filter through a dry, moderately retentive filter paper, discarding the first 75 ml.

6.2 Iodide Determination

6.2.1 Place 100 ml of pretreated sample (6.1) or a fraction thereof diluted to that volume, into a 150 ml beaker. Add a Teflon-coated stirring bar and place on a magnetic stirrer. Insert a Ph electrode and adjust the pH to approximately 7 or slightly less by the dropwise addition of H_2SO_4 solution (5.12).

6.2.2 Transfer the sample to a 250 ml widemouthed conical flask. Wash beaker with small amounts of distilled water and add washings to the flask. A 250 ml iodine flask would increase accuracy and precision by preventing possible loss of the iodine generated upon addition of potassium iodide and sulfuric acid (6.4.1).

6.2.3 Add 15 ml sodium acetate solution (5.8) and 5 ml acetic acid solution (5.1). Mix well. Add 40 ml bromine water solution (5.2): mix well. Wait 5 minutes.

6.2.4 Add 2 ml sodium formate solution (5.10); mix well. Wait 5 minutes.

6.2.5 Purge space above sample with gentle stream of nitrogen (5.21) for approximately 30 seconds to remove bromine fumes.

6.2.6 If a precipitate forms (iron), add 0.5 g KF·2H₂O (5.22).

6.2.7. A distilled water blank must be run with each set of samples because of iodide in reagents. If the blank is consistently shown to be zero for a particular "lot" of chemicals, it can be ignored.

6.2.8 Proceed to step (6.4).

6.3 Bromide Plus Iodide Determination

6.3.1 Place 100 ml of pretreated sample (6.1) or a fraction thereof diluted to that volume, in a 150 ml beaker. Add 5 g NaCl and stir to dissolve. Neutralize by dropwise addition of HCl solution (5.6) as in (6.2.1). Transfer as in (6.2.2).

6.3.2 Add 20 ml of calcium hypochlorite solution (5.4). Add 1 ml of HCl solution (5.6) and add approximately 0.2 g calcium carbonate (5.3).

6.3.3 Heat to boiling on a hot plate; maintain boiling for 8 minutes.

6.3.4 Remove from hot plate and carefully add 4 ml sodium formate solution (5.10). *Caution: Too rapid addition may cause foaming.* Wash down sides with distilled water.

6.3.5 Return to hot plate and maintain boiling conditions for an additional 8 minutes. Occasionally wash down sides with distilled water if residue is deposited from boiling action.

6.3.6 Remove from hot plate. Wash down sides and allow to cool.

6.3.7 If a precipitate forms (iron), add 0.5 g KF·2H₂O (5.22).

6.3.8 Add 3 drops sodium molybdate solution (5.11).

6.3.9 A distilled water blank must be run with each set of samples because of iodide, iodate, bromide, and/or bromate in reagents.

6.3.10 Proceed to step (6.4).

6.4 Titration

6.4.1 Dissolve approximately 1 g potassium iodide (5.7) in sample from (6.2.8 or 6.3.10). Add 10 ml of H₂SO₄ solution (5.12) and place in dark for 5 minutes.

6.4.2 Titrate with standardized phenylarsine oxide working standard (5.14) or sodium thiosulfate working standard (5.18), adding indicator (5.15, or 5.20) as end point is approached (light straw color). Titrate to colorless solution. Disregard returning blue color.

7. Calculations

7.1 Principle: Iodide is determined by the titration of the sample as oxidized in (6.2): bromide plus iodide is determined by the titration of the sample as oxidized in (6.3). The amount of bromide is then determined by difference. The number of equivalents of iodine produced a constant of 13,320 as shown in the equation in (7.2). Experimental data is entered in the appropriate place and the equation is solved for mg/1 bromide.

7.2 Equation

$$Br(mg/l) = 13{,}320 \left[\left(\frac{A \times B}{C} \right) - \left(\frac{D \times E}{F} \right) \right]$$

where

A = the number of ml of PAO needed to titrate the sample for bromide plus iodide (with the number of ml of

PAO needed to titrate the blank subtracted).

B = the normality of the PAO needed to titrate the sample for bromide plus iodide.

C = the volume of sample taken (100 ml or a fraction thereof) to be titrated for bromide plus iodide.

D = the number of ml of PAO needed to titrate the sample for iodide (with the number of ml of PAO needed to titrate the blank subtracted). The blank for the iodide titration is often zero.

E = the normality of the PAO used to titrate the sample for iodide.

F = the volume of sample taken (100 ml or a fraction thereof) to be titrated for iodide.

8. Precision and Accuracy

8.1 In a single laboratory (MDQARL), using a mixed domestic and industrial waste effluent, at concentrations of 0.3, 2.8, 5.3, 10.3 and 20.3 mg/l of bromide, the standard deviations were ±0.13, ±0.37, ±0.38, ±0.44 and ±0.42 mg/l, respectively.

8.2 In a single laboratory (MDQARL), using a mixed domestic and industrial waste effluent, at concentrations of 2.8, 5.3, 10.3 and 20.3 mg/l of bromide, recoveries were 96, 83, 97 and 99%, respectively.

Bibliography

1. ASTM Standards, Part 23, Water; Atmospheric Analysis, p 331–333, Method D1246-C (1973).

III. ORGANIC COMPOUNDS

Method for Benzidine and Its Salts in Water and Wastewater*

1. Scope and Application

1.1 This method covers the determination for benzidine and its salts in water and wastewaters. The method can be modified to apply also to the determination of closely related materials as described under Interferences (4.2).

1.2 The salts of benzidine, such as benzidine sulfate, are measured and reported as benzidine.

1.3 The method detection limit is 0.2 μg/l when analyzing 1 liter of sample.

2. Summary

2.1 The water sample is made basic and the benzidine is extracted with ethyl acetate. Cleanup is accomplished by extracting the benzidine from the ethyl acetate with hydrochloric acid. Chloramine-T is added to the acid solution to oxidize the benzidine. The yellow oxidation product is extracted with ethyl acetate and measured with a scanning spectrophotometer. The spectrum from 510 nm to 370 nm is used for qualitative identification.

3. Hazards

3.1 Benzidine is a known carcinogen. All manipulations of this method should be carried out in a hood with protection provided for the hands and arms of the analyst. Consult OSHA regulations (1) before working with benzidine.

---

*"Methods for Benzidine, Chlorinated Organic Compounds, Pentachlorophenol and Pesticides in Water and Wastewater" (INTERIM, Pending Issuance of Methods for Organic Analysis of Water and Wastes, September 1978), Environmental Protection Agency, Environmental Monitoring and Support Laboratory (EMSL).

4. Interferences

4.1 The multiple extractions effectively limit the interferences to organic bases. The oxidation with Chloramine-T to form a yellow product is very selective and has been described in detail (2,3). The use of the absorption spectrum for the identification of benzidine results in a highly specific procedure.

4.2 Some compounds having a structure very similar to benzidine will interfere with the quantification, if present. Examples of these interfering compounds are dichlorobenzidine, o-tolidine, and dianisidine.

4.3 A general yellow background color in the extract will limit the cell pathlength that can be employed and thus limit the sensitivity of the method.

5. Apparatus and Materials

5.1 Spectrophotometer-visible, scanning (510–370 nm).

5.2 Separatory Funnels — 125 ml, 250 ml, 2000 ml.

5.3 Cells — 1 to 5 cm pathlength, 20 ml volume maximum.

6. Reagents, Solvents and Standards

6.1 Ethyl acetate

6.2 Hydrochloric acid (1 N) — Add 83 ml conc. hydrochloric acid to water and dilute to one liter.

6.3 Chloramine-T — 10% solution. Prepare fresh daily by dissolving 1.0 g Chloramine-T in 10 ml distilled water.

6.4 Stock standard (0.2 μg/μl) — Dissolve 100.0 mg purified benzidine in about 30 ml 1 N HCl. Dilute to 500 ml with water.

7. Preparation of Calibration Curve

7.1 To a series of 125-ml separatory funnels, add 45 ml of hydrochloric acid and 10 ml of ethyl acetate. Shake for one minute to saturate the acid layers. Discard the solvent layers. Dose the series with volumes from 1.0 to 20.0 μl of stock standard, using syringes.

7.2 Treat standards according to the Procedure beginning with 9.5.

8. Quality Control

8.1 Duplicate and spiked sample analyses are recommended as quality control checks. Quality control charts should be developed and used as a check on the analytical system. Quality control check samples and performance evaluation samples should be analyzed on a regular basis.

8.2 Each time a set of samples is extracted, a method blank is determined on a volume of distilled water equivalent to that used to dilute the sample.

9. Procedure

9.1 Adjust the sample pH to 8.5 to 9.0 with dilute NaOH or HCl.

9.2 Transfer 1 liter of sample to a 2000-ml separatory funnel. Add 150 ml ethyl acetate and shake for two minutes. Allow the layers to separate, then drain the water layer into a second 2-liter separatory funnel. Drain the solvent layer into a 250-ml separatory funnel.

9.3 Repeat the extraction of the water layer twice more with 50-ml portions of ethyl acetate. Combine all solvent layers, then discard the water layer.

9.4 Extract the solvent layer three times with 15-ml portions of hydrochloric acid by shaking 2 minutes and allowing the phases to separate. Combine the acid layers in a glass stoppered container for cold storage until time is available for anal-

ysis, or transfer the layers directly into a 125-ml separatory funnel.

9.5 Prepare the spectrophotometer so it is warmed and ready to use. The remaining steps of the procedure must be performed rapidly on one sample at a time.

9.6 To the hydrochloric acid solution in a 125 ml separatory funnel, add 1.0 ml chloramine-T solution and mix. Add 25.0 ml ethyl acetate with a pipet and shake for two minutes. Allow the layers to separate, then discard the aqueous phase.

9.7 Filter the solvent layer through coarse filter paper and fill a 5-cm cell with the filtrate.

9.8 Scan the solvent from 510 nm to 370 nm. Ethyl acetate is used for a blank with double beam instruments. Shorter pathlength cells should be used in cases where absorbance exceeds 0.8.

10. Calculation of Results

10.1 Benzidine is identified by its absorbance maximum at 436 nm. Dichlorobenzidine gives similar response but has its absorbance maximum at 445 nm.

10.2 Construct a baseline from the absorbance minimum at about 470 nm to the minimum at 390 nm (or 420 nm minimum for samples with a high background). Record the absorbance of the peak maximum and the absorbance of the constructed baseline at the 436 nm. Treat samples and standards in the same fashion.

10.3 Using the net absorbance values, prepare a calibration plot from the standards. Determine the total micrograms in each sample from this plot.

10.4 Divide the total micrograms by the sample volume, in liters, to determine μg/l. Correct results for cell pathlength if necessary.

11. Reporting Results

11.1 Report results in micrograms per liter as benzidine without correction for recovery data. When duplicate and spike samples are analyzed all data obtained should be reported.

12. Accuracy and Precision

12.1 When 1 liter samples of river water were dosed with 1.80 μg of benzidine, an average of 1.24 μg was recovered. The standard deviation was 0.092 μg/l (n = 8).

References

1. *Federal Register*, Volume 39, Page 3779, Paragraph 1910.93; (January 29, 1974).
2. Glassman, J. M., and Meigs, J. W., "Benzidine (4,4'-Diaminobiphenyl) and Substituted Benzidines", *Arch. Industr. Hyg., 4,* 519, (1951).
3. Butt, L. T., and Strafford, N., "Papilloma of the Bladder in the Chemical Industry. Analytical Methods for the Determination of Benzidine and B-Naphtylamine, Recommended by A.B.C.M. Sub-Committee", *J. Appl. Chem., 6,* 525 (1956).

Method for Pentachlorophenol in Water and Wastewater*

1. Scope and Application

1.1 This method covers the determination of pentachlorophenol (PCP) in water and wastewater.

2. Summary

2.1 Pentachlorophenol is extracted from the acidified water sample (pH 3) with toluene, methylated with diazomethane, and analyzed by electron-capture gas chromatography, using the columns listed in the organochlorine pesticide method. (Page 7, EPA manual*; *Standard Methods* 15th edition, p. 493).

2.2 Further identification of pentachlorophenol is made with a mass spectrometer.

---

*"Methods for Benzidine, Chlorinated Organic Compounds, Pentachlorophenol and Pesticides in Water and Wastewater" (INTERIM, Pending Issuance of Methods for Organic Analysis of Water and Wastes, September 1978), Environmental Protection Agency, Environmental Monitoring and Support Laboratory (EMSL). Text of method in this source is complete as given above.

3. Interferences

3.1 Chlorinated pesticides and other high boiling chlorinated organic compounds may interfere with the analysis of PCP.

3.2 Injections of samples not treated with diazomethane indicate, to a certain degree, whether interfering substances are present.

4. Precision and Accuracy

4.1 Single laboratory accuracy and precision reported for this method when analyzing five replicates of tap water spiked with 0.05 to 0.07 μg/l of PCP is as follows:

Recovery—mean 95.9%, range 88.1 to 100.2%

Standard Deviation—6.0%

Reference:

1. "Analysis of Pentachlorophenol Residues in Soil, Water and Fish," Stark, A., Agricultural and Food Chemistry, *17*, 871 (July/August 1969).

Method for Organophosphorus Pesticides in Water and Wastewater*

1. Scope and Application

1.1 This method covers the determination of various organophosphorus pesticides in water and wastewater.

1.2 The following pesticides may be determined individually by this method:

Azinphos methyl
Demeton-O
Demeton-S
Diazinon
Disulfoton
Malathion
Parathion methyl
Parathion ethyl

2. Summary

2.1 The method offers several analytical alternatives, dependent on the analyst's assessment of the nature and extent of interferences and the complexity of the pesticide mixtures found. Specifically, the procedure describes the use of an effective co-solvent for efficient sample extraction; provides, through use of the column chromatography and liquid-liquid partition, methods for the elimination of non-pesticide interferences and the preseparation of pesticide mixtures. Identification is made by selective gas chromatographic separation and may be corroborated through the use of two or more unlike columns. Detection and measurement are best accomplished by flame photometric gas chromatography using a phosphorus specific filter. The electron capture detector, though non-specific, may also be used

for those compounds to which it responds. Results are reported in micrograms per liter.

2.2 Confirmation of the identity of the compounds should be made by GC-MS when a new or undefined sample type is being analyzed and the concentration is adequate for such determination.

2.3 This method is recommended for use only by experienced pesticide analysts or under the close supervision of such qualified persons.

3. Interferences

3.1 Solvents, reagents, glassware, and other sample processing hardware may yield discrete artifacts and/or elevated baselines, causing misinterpretation of gas chromatograms. All of these materials must be demonstrated to be free from interferences under the conditions of the analysis. Specific selection of reagents and purification of solvents by distillation in all-glass systems may be required. Refer to Appendix I.* †

3.2 The interferences in industrial effluents are high and varied and often pose great difficulty in obtaining accurate and precise measurement of organophosphorus pesticides. Sample clean-up procedures are generally required and may result in the loss of certain organophosphorus pesticides. Therefore, great care should be exercised in the selection and use of methods for eliminating or minimizing interferences. It is not possible to describe procedures for overcoming all of the interferences that may be encountered in industrial effluents.

3.3 Compounds such as organochlorine pesticides, polychlorinated biphenyls and

---

* "Methods for Benzidine, Chlorinated Organic Compounds, Pentachlorophenol and Pesticides in Water and Wastewater" (INTERIM, Pending Issuance of Methods for Organic Analysis of Water and Wastes, September 1978), Environmental Protection Agency, Environmental Monitoring and Support Laboratory (EMSL).

† Reproduced below.

phthalate esters interfere with the analysis of organophosphorus pesticides by electron capture gas chromatography. When encountered, these interferences are overcome by the use of the phosphorus specific flame photometric detector. If such a detector is not available, these interferences may be removed from the sample by using the clean-up procedures described in the EPA methods for those compounds (1, 2).

3.4 Elemental sulfur will interfere with the determination of organophosphorus pesticides by flame photometric and electron capture gas chromatography. The elimination of elemental sulfur as an interference is described in Section 10.5, Cleanup and Separation Procedures.

4. Apparatus and Materials

4.1 Gas Chromatograph—Equipped with glass lined injection port.

4.2 Detector options:

4.2.1 Flame Photometric—526 mu phosphorus filter.

4.2.2 Electron Capture—Radioactive (tritium or nickel-63).

4.3 Recorder—Potentiometric strip chart (10 in.) compatible with the detector.

4.4 Gas Chromatographic Column Materials:

4.4.1 Tubing—Pyrex (180 cm × 4 mm ID)

4.4.2 Glass Wool—Silanized

4.4.3 Solid Support—Gas Chrom Q (100–120 mesh)

4.4.4 Liquid Phases—Expressed as weight percent coated on solid support.

4.4.4.1 OV-1, 3%

4.4.4.2 OV-210, 5%

4.4.4.3 OV-17, 1.5% plus QF-1 or OV-210, 1.95%

4.4.4.4 QF-1 or OV-210, 6% plus SE-30, 4%

4.5 Kuderna-Danish (K-D) Glassware

4.5.1 Snyder Column—three ball (macro) and two ball (micro)

4.5.2 Evaporative Flasks—500 ml

4.5.3 Receiver Ampuls—10 ml, graduated

4.5.4 Ampul Stoppers

4.6 Chromatographic Column—Chromaflex (400 mm × 19 mm ID) with coarse fritted plate and Teflon stopcock on bottom; 250 ml reservoir bulb at top of column with flared out funnel shape at top of bulb—a special order (Kontes K-420540-9011).

4.7 Chromatographic Column—pyrex (approximately 400 mm long × 20 mm ID) with coarse fritted plate on bottom.

4.8 Micro Syringes—10, 25, 50 and 100 μl.

4.9 Separatory funnels—125 ml, 1000 ml and 2000 ml with Teflon stopcock.

4.10 Micro-pipets—disposable (140 mm long × 5 mm ID).

4.11 Blender—High speed, glass or stainless steel cup.

4.12 Graduated cylinders—100 and 250 ml.

4.13 Florisil—PR Grade (60–100 mesh); purchase activated at 1250° F and store in the dark in glass containers with glass stoppers or foil-lined screw caps. Before use, activate each batch overnight at 130° C in foil-covered glass containers. Determine lauric-acid value (See Appendix II).* ‡

4.14 Alumina—Woelm, neutral; deactivate by pipeting 1 ml of distilled water into 125 ml ground glass-stoppered Erlenmeyer flask. Rotate flask to distribute

---

* "Methods for Benzidine, Chlorinated Organic Compounds, Pentachlorophenol and Pesticides in Water and Wastewater" (INTERIM, Pending Issuance of Methods for Organic Analysis of Water and Wastes, September 1978), Environmental Protection Agency, Environmental Monitoring and Support Laboratory (EMSL).

‡ Also given as Appendix to Section 509A, p. 501, *Standard Methods,* 15th edition.

water over surface of glass. Immediately add 19.0 g fresh alumina through small powder funnel. Shake flask containing mixture for two hours on a mechanical shaker (3).

5. Reagents, Solvents, and Standards

5.1 Sodium Chloride—(ACS) Saturated solution in distilled water (pre-rinse NaCl with hexane).

5.2 Sodium Hydroxide—(ACS) 10 N in distilled water.

5.3 Sodium Sulfate—(ACS) Granular, anhydrous (conditioned at 400° C for 4 hrs.).

5.4 Sulfuric Acid—(ACS) Mix equal volumes of conc. H_2SO_4 with distilled water.

5.5 Diethyl Ether—Nanograde, redistilled in glass, if necessary.

5.5.1 Must be free of peroxides as indicated by EM Quant test strips. (Test strips are available from EM Laboratories, Inc., 500 Executive Blvd., Elmsford, N.Y. 10523.)

5.5.2 Procedures recommended for removal of peroxides are provided with the test strips.

5.6 Acetonitrile, Hexane, Methanol, Methylene Chloride, Petroleum Ether (boiling range 30–60° C)—nanograde, redistill in glass if necessary.

5.7 Pesticide Standards—Reference grade.

6. Calibration

6.1 Gas chromatographic operating conditions are considered acceptable if the response to dicapthon is at least 50% of full scale when ≥1.5 ng is injected for flame photometric detection and ≥0.06 ng is injected for electron capture detection. For all quantitative measurements, the detector must be operated within its linear re-

sponse range and the detector noise level should be less than 2% of full scale.

6.2 Standards are injected frequently as a check on the stability of operating conditions. Gas chromatograms of several standard pesticides are shown in Figures 1, 2, 3 and 4 and provide reference operating conditions for the four recommended columns.

6.3 The elution order and retention ratios of various organophosphorus pesticides are provided in Table 1, as a guide.

7. Quality Control

7.1 Duplicate and spiked sample analyses are recommended as quality control checks. Quality control charts (4) should be developed and used as a check on the analytical system. Quality control check samples and performance evaluation samples should be analyzed on a regular basis.

7.2 Each time a set of samples is ex-

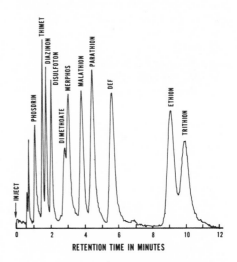

Figure 1. Column Packing: 1.5% OV-17 + 1.95% QF-1, Carrier Gas: Nitrogen at 70 ml/min, Column Temperature: 215 C, Detector: Flame Photometric (Phosphorus).

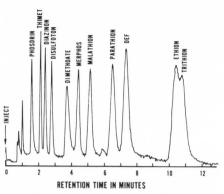

Figure 3. Column Packing: 6% QF-1 + 4% SE-30, Carrier Gas: Nitrogen at 70 ml/min, Column Temperature: 215C, Detector: Flame Photometric (Phosphorus).

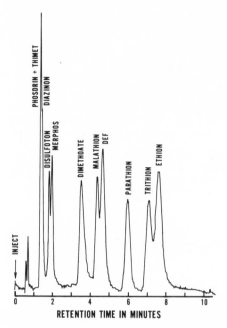

Figure 2. Column Packing: 5% OV-210, Carrier Gas: Nitrogen at 60 ml/min, Column Temperature: 200 C, Detector: Flame Photometric (Phosphorus).

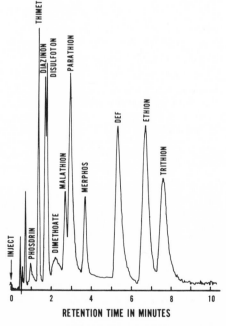

Figure 4. Column Packing: 3% OV-1, Carrier Gas: Nitrogen at 60 ml/min, Column Temperature: 200 C, Detector: Flame Photometric (Phosphorus).

tracted, a method blank is determined on a volume of distilled water equivalent to that used to dilute the sample.

8. Sample Preparation

8.1 The sample size taken for analysis is dependent on the type of sample and the sensitivity required for the purpose at hand. Background information on the pesticide levels previously detected at a given sampling site will assist in determining the sample size required, as well as the final volume to which the extract needs to be concentrated. A 1-liter sample is usually taken for drinking water and ambient water analysis to provide a detection limit of 0.050 to 0.100 μg/l. One-hundred milliliters is usually adequate to provide a

TABLE 1. RETENTION TIMES OF SOME ORGANOPHOSPHORUS PESTICIDES RELATIVE TO PARATHION

Liquid Phase[1]	1.5% OV-17 + 1.95% QF-1[2]	6% QF-1[2] + 4% SE-30	5% OV-210	7% OV-1
Column Temp.	215 C	215 C	200 C	200 C
Nitrogen Carrier Flow	70 ml/min	70 ml/min	60 ml/min	60 ml/min
Pesticide	RR	RR	RR	RR
Demeton[3]	0.46	0.26	0.20	0.74
		0.43	0.38	
Diazinon	0.40	0.38	0.25	0.59
Disulfoton	0.46	0.45	0.31	0.62
Malathion	0.86	0.78	0.73	0.92
Parathion methyl	0.82	0.80	0.81	0.79
Parathion ethyl	1.00	1.00	1.00	1.00
Azinphos methyl	6.65	4.15	4.44	4.68
Parathion (min absolute)	4.5	6.6	5.7	3.1

[1] All columns glass, 180 cm × 4 mm ID, solid support Gas-Chrom Q, 100/120 mesh.
[2] May substitute OV-210 for QF-1.
[3] Anomalous, multipeak response often encountered.

detection limit of 1 μg/l for industrial effluents.

8.2 Quantitatively transfer the proper aliquot of sample from the sample container into a two-liter separatory funnel. If less than 800 ml is analyzed, dilute to one liter with interference free distilled water.

9. Extraction

9.1 Add 60 ml of 15% methylene chloride in hexane (v:v) to the sample in the separatory funnel and shake vigorously for two minutes.

9.2 Allow the mixed solvent to separate from the sample, then draw the water into a one-liter Erlenmeyer flask. Pour the organic layer into a 100 ml beaker and then pass it through a column containing 3–4 inches of anhydrous sodium sulfate, and collect it in a 500 ml K-D flask equipped with a 10 ml ampul. Return the water phase to the separatory funnel. Rinse the Erlenmeyer flask with a second 60 ml volume of solvent; add the solvent to the separatory funnel and complete the extrac-

tion procedure a second time. Perform a third extraction in the same manner.

9.3 Concentrate the extract in the K-D evaporator on a hot water bath.

9.4 Analyze by gas chromatography unless a need for clean-up is indicated. (See Section 10).

10. Clean-up and Separation Procedures

10.1 Interferences in the form of distinct peaks and/or high background in the initial gas chromatographic analysis, as well as the physical characteristics of the extract (color, cloudiness, viscosity) and background knowledge of the sample source will indicate whether clean-up is required. When these interfere with measurement of the pesticides, or affect column life or detector sensitivity, proceed as directed below. The use of these procedures is not required for samples free of interferences. They are provided as options to the analyst to be used when needed.

10.2 Acetonitrile Partition—This procedure is used to separate fats and oils from the sample extracts. It should be noted that not all pesticides are quantitatively recovered by this procedure. The analyst must be aware of this and demonstrate the efficiency of the partitioning for specific pesticides.

10.2.1 Quantitatively transfer the previously concentrated extract to a 125-ml separatory funnel with enough hexane to bring the final volume to 15 ml. Extract the sample four times by shaking vigorously for one minute with 30 ml portions of hexane-saturated acetonitrile.

10.2.2 Combine and transfer the acetonitrile phases to a one-liter separatory funnel and add 650 ml of distilled water and 40 ml of saturated sodium chloride solution. Mix thoroughly for 30–45 seconds. Extract with two 100 ml portions of hexane by vigorously shaking about 15 seconds.

10.2.3 Combine the hexane extracts in a one-liter separatory funnel and wash with two 100 ml portions of distilled water. Discard the water layer and pour the hexane layer through a 3–4 inch anhydrous sodium sulfate column into a 500-ml K-D flask equipped with a 10-ml ampul. Rinse the separatory funnel and column with three 10 ml portions of hexane.

10.2.4 Concentrate the extracts to 6–10 ml in the K-D evaporator in a hot water bath.

10.2.5 Analyze by gas chromatography unless a need for further clean-up is indicated.

10.3 Florisil   Column   Adsorption Chromatography

10.3.1 Adjust the sample extract volume to 10 ml.

10.3.2 Place a charge of activated Florisil (weight determined by lauric-acid value, see Appendix II* ‡) in a Chromaflex column. After settling the Florisil by tapping the column, add about one-half inch layer of anhydrous granular sodium sulfate to the top.

10.3.3 Pre-elute the column, after cooling, with 50–60 ml of petroleum ether. Discard the eluate and just prior to exposure of the sulfate layer to air, quantitatively transfer the sample extract into the column by decantation and subsequent petroleum ether washings. Adjust the elution rate to about 5 ml per minute and, separately, collect up to four eluates in 500-ml K-D flasks equipped with 10-ml ampuls. (See Eluate Composition, 10.4.) Perform the first elution with 200 ml of 6% ethyl ether in petroleum ether, and the second elution with 200 ml of 15% ethyl ether in petroleum ether. Perform the third elution with 200 ml of 50% ethyl ether—petroleum ether and the fourth elution with 200 ml of 100% ethyl ether.

10.3.4 Concentrate the eluates to 6-10 ml in the K-D evaporator in a hot water bath.

10.3.5 Analyze by gas chromatography.

10.4 Eluate Composition—By using an equivalent quantity of any batch of Florisil as determined by its lauric-acid value, the pesticides will be separated into the eluates indicated below:

6% Eluate	15% Eluate
Demeton	Diazinon
Disulfoton	Malathion (trace)
	Parathion Methyl

---

* "Methods for Benzidine, Chlorinated Organic Compounds, Pentachlorophenol and Pesticides in Water and Wastewater" (INTERIM, Pending Issuance of Methods for Organic Analysis of Water and Wastes, September 1978), Environmental Protection Agency, Environmental Monitoring and Support Laboratory (EMSL).

‡ Also given as Appendix to Section 509A, p. 501, *Standard Methods,* 15th edition.

50% Eluate	100% Eluate
Malathion	Azinphos methyl
Azinphos methyl	(80%)
(20%)	

For additional information regarding eluate composition, refer to the FDA Pesticide Analytical Manual (5).

10.5 Removal of Sulfur—If elemental sulfur interferes with the gas chromatographic analysis, it can be removed by the use of an alumina microcolumn.

10.5.1 Adjust the sample extract volume to 0.5 ml in a K-D apparatus, using a two-ball Snyder microcolumn.

10.5.2 Plug a disposable pipet with a small quantity of glass wool. Add enough alumina to produce a 3-cm column after settling. Top the alumina with a 0.5-cm layer of anhydrous sodium sulfate.

10.5.3 Quantitatively transfer the concentrated extract to the alumina microcolumn using a 100 μl syringe. Rinse the ampul with 200 μl of hexane and add to the microcolumn.

10.5.4 Elute the microcolumn with 3 ml of hexane and discard the first eluate which contains the elemental sulfur.

10.5.5 Next elute the column with 5 ml of 10% hexane in methylene chloride. Collect the eluate in a 10 ml graduated ampul.

10.5.6 Analyze by gas chromatography.

NOTE: If the electron capture detector is to be used methylene chloride must be removed. To do this, attach the ampul to a K-D apparatus (500-ml flask and 3-ball Snyder column) and concentrate to about 0.5 ml. Adjust volume as required prior to analysis.

11. Calculation of Results

11.1 Determine the pesticide concentration by using the absolute calibration procedure described below or the relative calibration procedure described in Appendix III.* †

$$(1) \quad \text{Micrograms/liter} = \frac{(A) \ (B) \ (V_t)}{(V_i) \ (V_s)}$$

$$A = \frac{\text{ng standard}}{\text{Standard area}}$$

B = Sample aliquot area
V_i = Volume of extract injected (μl)
V_t = Volume of total extract (μl)
V_s = Volume of water extracted (ml)

12. Reporting Results

12.1 Report results in micrograms per liter without correction for recovery data. When duplicate and spiked samples are analyzed all data obtained should be reported.

References

1. "Method for Chlorinated Hydrocarbons in Water and Wastewater", EPA Interim Methods, Sept. 1978, p. 7.
2. "Method for Polychlorinated Biphenyls (PCBs) in Water and Wastewater", EPA Interim Methods, Sept. 1978, p. 43.
3. Law, L. M. and Georlitz, D. F., "Microcolumn Chromatographic Clean-up for the Analysis of Pesticides in Water", *Journal of the Association for Analytical Chemists, 53*, 1276 (1970).
4. "Handbook for Analytical Quality Control in Water and Wastewater Laboratories", Chapter 6, Section 6.4, U. S. Environmental Protection Agency, National Environmental Research Center, Analytical Quality Control Laboratory, Cincinnati, Ohio, 45268, 1973.
5. "Pesticide Analytical Manual", U. S. Dept. of Health, Education and Welfare, Food and Drug Administration, Washington, D. C.

---

* "Methods for Benzidine, Chlorinated Organic Compounds, Pentachlorophenol and Pesticides in Water and Wastewater" (INTERIM, Pending Issuance of Methods for Organic Analysis of Water and Wastes, September 1978), Environmental Protection Agency, Environmental Monitoring and Support Laboratory (EMSL).

† Reproduced below.

APPENDIX I
CONSIDERATIONS FOR GLASSWARE AND REAGENTS
USED IN ORGANIC ANALYSIS*

1. Glassware

1.1 Cleaning Procedure—It is particularly important that glassware used in trace organic analyses be scrupulously cleaned before initial use as well as after each analysis. The glassware should be cleaned as soon as possible after use, first rinsing with water or the solvent that was last used in it. This should be followed by washing with hot soap water, rinsing with tap water, distilled water, redistilled acetone and finally with pesticide quality hexane. Heavily contaminated glassware may require muffling at 400°C for 15- to 30-minutes. High boiling materials, such as some of the polychlorinated biphenyls (PCBs) may not be eliminated by such heat treatment. NOTE: Volumetric ware should not be muffled. The glassware should be stored immediately after drying to prevent accumulation of dust or other contaminants. Store inverted or cover mouth with foil.

1.2 Calibration—Individual Kuderna-Danish concentrator tubes and/or centrifuge tubes used for final concentration of extracts must be accurately calibrated at the working volume. This is especially important at volumes below 1 ml. Calibration should be made using a precision microsyringe, recording the volume required to bring the liquid level to the individual graduation marks. Glass A volumetric ware should be used for preparing all standard solutions.

2. Standards, Reagents and Solvents

2.1 Analytical Standards and Other Chemicals—Analytical reference grade standards should be used whenever available. They should be stored according to the manufacturer's instructions. Standards and reagents sensitive to light should be stored in dark bottles and/or in a cool dark place. Those requiring refrigeration should be allowed to come to room temperature before opening. Storing of such standards under nitrogen is advisable.

2.1.1 Stock Standards—Pesticide stock standards solutions should be prepared in 1 μg/μl concentrations by dissolving 0.100-grams of the standard in pesticide-quality hexane or other appropriate solvent (Acetone should not be used since some pesticides degrade on standing in this solvent) and diluting to volume in a 100 ml ground glass stoppered volumetric flask. The stock solution is transferred to ground glass stoppered reagent bottles. These standards should be checked frequently for signs of degradation and concentration, especially just prior to preparing working standards from them.

2.1.2 Working Standards—Pesticide working standards are prepared from the stock solutions using a micro syringe preferably equipped with a Chaney adapter. The concentration of the working standards will vary depending on the detection system employed and the level of pesticide in the samples to be analyzed. A typical concentration (0.1 ng/μl) may be prepared by diluting 1 μl of the 1 μg/μl stock to volume in a 10-ml ground glass stoppered volumetric flask. The standard solutions should be transferred to ground glass stop-

---

*"Methods for Organic Pesticides in Water and Wastewater," 1971, Environmental Protection Agency, National Environmental Research Center, Cincinnati, Ohio, 45268.

pered reagent bottles. Preparation of a fresh working standard each day will minimize concentration through evaporation of solvent. These standards should be stored in the same manner as the stock solutions.

2.1.3 Identification of Reagents—All stock and working standards should be labeled as follows: name of compound, concentration, date prepared, solvent used, and name of person who prepared it.

2.1.4 Anhydrous sodium sulfate used as a drying agent for solvent extracts should be prewashed with the solvent or solvents that it comes in contact with in order to remove any interferences that may be present.

2.1.5 Glass wool used at the top of the sodium sulfate column must be pre-extracted for about 40-hours in soxhlet using the appropriate solvent.

2.2 Solvents—Organic solvents must be of pesticide quality and demonstrated to be free of interferences in a manner compatible with whatever analytical operation is to be performed. Solvents can be checked by analyzing a volume equivalent to that used in the analysis and concentrated to the minimum final volume. Interferences are noted in terms of gas chromatographic response—relative retention time, peak geometry, peak intensity and width of solvent response. Interferences noted under these conditions can be considered maximum. If necessary, a solvent must be redistilled in glass using a high efficiency distillation system. A 60-cm column packed with ⅛ inch glass helices is effective.

2.2.1 Ethyl Ether—Hexane—It is particularly important that these two solvents, used for extraction of organochlorine pesticides from water, be checked for interferences just prior to use. Ethyl ether, in particular, can produce troublesome interferences. (NOTE: The formation of peroxides in ethyl ether creates a potential explosion hazard. Therefore it must be checked for peroxides before use.) It is recommended that the solvents be mixed just prior to use and only in the amount required for immediate use since build-up of interferences often occurs on standing.

2.2.2 The great sensitivity of the electron capture detector requires that all solvents used for the analysis be of pesticide quality. Even these solvents sometimes require redistillation in an all glass system prior to use. The quality of the solvents may vary from lot to lot and even within the same lot, so that each bottle of solvent must be checked before use.

APPENDIX III
CHROMATOGRAPHIC CALIBRATION TECHNIQUE

Relative Calibration (Internal Standardization):

A relative calibration curve is prepared by simultaneously chromatographing mixtures of the previously identified sample constituent and a reference standard in known weight ratios and plotting the weight ratios against area ratios. An accurately known amount of the reference material is then added to the sample and the mixture chromatographed. The area ratios are calculated and the weight ratio is read from the curve. Since the amount of reference material added is known, the amount of the sample constituent can be calculated as follows:

$$\text{micrograms/liter} = \frac{Rw \times Ws}{Vs}$$

Rw = Weight ratio of component to standard obtained from calibration curve

Ws = Weight of internal standard added to sample in nanograms

Vs = Volume of sample in milliliters

Using this method, injection volumes need not be accurately measured the detector response need not remain constant since changes in response will not alter the ratio. This method is preferred when the internal standard meets the following conditions:

a) well-resolved from other peaks
b) elutes close to peaks of interest
c) approximates concentration of unknown
d) structurally similar to unknown.

Method for O-Aryl Carbamate Pesticides in Water and Wastewater*

1. Scope and Application

1.1 This method covers the determination of various O-aryl carbamate pesticides in water and wastewater.

1.2 The following pesticides may be determined individually by this method:

Aminocarb
Carbaryl
Methiocarb
Mexacarbate
Propoxur

2. Summary

2.1 A measured volume of water is extracted with methylene chloride. The concentrated extract is cleaned up with a Florisil column. Appropriate fractions from the column are concentrated and portions are separated by thin-layer chromatog-

raphy. The carbamates are hydrolyzed on the layer and the hydrolysis products are reacted with 2,6-dibromoquinone chlorimide to yield specific colored products. Quantitative measurement is achieved by visually comparing the responses of sample extracts to the responses of standards on the same thin-layer. Identifications are confirmed by changing the pH of the layer and observing color changes of the reaction products. Results are reported in micrograms per liter.

2.2 This method is recommended for use only by experienced pesticide analysts or under the close supervision of such qualified persons.

3. Interferences

3.1 Direct interferences may be encountered from phenols that may be present in the sample. These materials react with the chromogenic reagent and yield reaction products similar to those of the carbamates. In cases where phenols are suspected of interfering with a determination, a different solvent system should be used to attempt to isolate the carbamates.

---

*"Methods for Benzidine, Chlorinated Organic Compounds, Pentachlorophenol and Pesticides in Water and Wastewater" (INTERIM, Pending Issuance of Methods for Organic Analysis of Water and Wastes, September 1978), Environmental Protection Agency, Environmental Monitoring and Support Laboratory (EMSL).

3.2 Indirect interferences may be encountered from naturally colored materials whose presence masks the chromogenic reaction.

4. Apparatus and Materials

4.1 Thin-layer plates—Glass plates (200 × 200 mm) coated with 0.25 mm layer of Silica Gel G (gypsum binder).

4.2 Spotting Template

4.3 Developing Chamber

4.4 Sprayer—20 ml capacity

4.5 Kuderna-Danish (K-D) Glassware (Kontes)

4.5.1 Snyder Column—three ball (K-503000)

4.5.2 Micro-Snyder Column—two ball (K-569001)

4.5.3 Evaporative Flasks—500 ml (K-570001)

4.5.4 Receiver Ampuls—10 ml graduated (K-570050)

4.5.5 Ampul Stoppers

4.6 Chromatographic Column—Chromaflex (400 mm long × 19 mm ID) with coarse fritted plate on bottom and Teflon stopcock; 250 ml reservoir bulb at top of column with flared out funnel shape at top of bulb—a special order (Kontes K-420540-9011).

4.7 Chromatographic Column—Pyrex (approximately 400 mm long × 20 mm ID) with coarse fritted plate on bottom.

4.8 Micro Syringes—10, 25, 50 and 100 µl.

4.9 Separatory Funnel—2000 ml, with Teflon stopcock.

4.10 Blender—High speed, glass or stainless steel cup.

4.11 Florisil—PR Grade (60–80 mesh); purchase activated at 1250° F and store in the dark in glass containers with glass stoppers or foil-lined screw caps. Before use activate each batch overnight at 130° C in foil-covered glass container. Determine lauric acid value (see Appendix II)* †.

5. Reagents, Solvents, and Standards

5.1 Sodium Hydroxide—(ACS) 10 N in distilled water.

5.2 Sodium Sulfate—(ACS) Granular, anhydrous.

5.3 Sulfuric Acid—(ACS) Mix equal volumes of conc. H_2SO_4 with distilled water.

5.4 Diethyl Ether—Nanograde, redistilled in glass, if necessary.

5.4.1 Must be free of peroxides as indicated by EM Quant test strips. (Test strips are available from EM Laboratories, Inc., 500 Executive Blvd., Elmsford, N.Y. 10523.)

5.4.2 Procedures recommended for removal of peroxides are provided with the test strips.

5.5 Hexane, Methanol, Methylene Chloride, Petroleum Ether—nanograde, redistill in glass if necessary.

5.6 Pesticide Standards—Reference grade.

5.6.1 TLC Standards—0.100 µg/µl in chloroform.

5.7 Chromogenic agent—Dissolve 0.2 g 2,6-dibromoquinone chlorimide in 20 ml chloroform.

5.8 Buffer solution—0.1 N sodium borate in water.

6. Calibration

6.1 To insure even solvent travel up the layer, the tank used for layer development must be thoroughly saturated with devel-

---

* "Methods for Benzidine, Chlorinated Organic Compounds, Pentachlorophenol and Pesticides in Water and Wastewater" (INTERIM, Pending Issuance of Methods for Organic Analysis of Water and Wastes, September 1978), Environmental Protection Agency, Environmental Monitoring and Support Laboratory (EMSL).

† Also given as Appendix to Section 509A, p. 501, *Standard Methods*, 15th edition.

TABLE 1. R$_f$ VALUES OF O-ARYL CARBAMATE PESTICIDES IN SEVERAL SOLVENT SYSTEMS

	A	B	C	D	E	F
Carbaryl	0.26	0.22	0.48	0.41	0.58	0.24
Aminocarb	0.26	0.02	0.46	0.52	0.54	0.04
Mexacarbate	0.34	0.22	0.54	0.53	0.60	0.24
Methiocarb	0.31	0.31	0.55	0.55	0.59	0.28
Propoxur	0.27	0.10	0.53	0.59	0.60	0.13

Solvent Systems: A. Hexane/acetone (3:1); B. Methylene chloride; C. Benzene/acetone (4:1); D. Benzene/cyclohexane/diethylamine (5:2:2); E. Ethyl acetate; F. Chloroform.

oping solvent before it is used. This may be achieved by lining the inner walls of the tank with chromatography paper and introducing the solvent 1–2 hours before use.

6.2 Samples and standards should be introduced to the layer using a syringe, micropipet or other suitable device that permits all the spots to be about the same size and as small as possible. An air stream directed on the layer during spotting will speed solvent evaporation and help to maintain small spots.

6.3 For qualitative and quantitative work, spot a series representing 0.1–1.0 μg of a pesticide. Tables 1 and 2 present color responses and R$_f$ values for several solvent systems.

7. Quality Control

7.1 Duplicate and spiked sample anal-

TABLE 2. COLOR RESPONSES AND DETECTION LIMIT FOR O-ARYL CARBAMATES

	Colors		Detection
	Before Buffer	After Buffer	Limit (μg)
Carbaryl	Brown	Red-Purple	0.1
Aminocarb	Gray	Green	0.1
Mexacarbate	Gray	Green	0.1
Methiocarb	Brown	Tan	0.2
Propoxur	Blue	Blue	0.1

yses are recommended as quality control checks. Quality control charts should be developed and used as a check on the analytical system. Quality control check samples and performance evaluation samples should be analyzed on a regular basis.

7.2 Each time a set of samples is extracted, a method blank is determined on a volume of distilled water equivalent to that used to dilute the sample.

8. Sample Preparation

8.1 Blend the sample if suspended matter is present and adjust pH to near neutral (pH 6.5–7.5) with 50% sulfuric acid or 10 N sodium hydroxide.

8.2 Quantitatively transfer a one-liter aliquot into a two-liter separatory funnel.

9. Extraction

9.1 Add 60 ml of methylene chloride to the sample in the separatory funnel and shake vigorously for two minutes.

9.2 Allow the solvent to separate from the sample, draw the organic layer into a 100-ml beaker, then pass the organic layer through a chromatographic column containing 3–4 inches anhydrous sodium sulfate, and collect it in a 500-ml K-D flask equipped with a 10-ml ampul. Add a second 60-ml volume of solvent to the separatory funnel and complete the extraction procedure a second time. Perform a third extraction in the same manner.

9.3 Concentrate the extract to 10 ml in a K-D evaporator on a hot water bath. Disconnect the Snyder column just long enough to add 10 ml of hexane to the K-D flask and then continue the concentration to about 5–6 ml. If the need for cleanup is indicated, continue to Florisil Column Cleanup (10 below).

9.4 If further cleanup is not required, replace the Snyder column and flask with a micro-Snyder column and continue the concentration to 0.5–1.0 ml. Analyze this final concentrate by thin-layer chromatography (Section 11).

10. Florisil Column Cleanup

10.1 Adjust the sample extract to 10 ml with hexane.

10.2 Place a charge of activated Florisil (weight determined by lauric-acid value, see Appendix II* †) in a Chromaflex column. After settling the Florisil by tapping the column, add about one-half inch layer of anhydrous granular sodium sulfate to the top.

10.3 Pre-elute the column, after cooling, with 50–60 ml of petroleum ether. Discard the eluate and just prior to exposure of the sulfate layer to air, quantitatively transfer the sample extract into the column by decantation and subsequent petroleum ether washings. Adjust the elution rate to about 5 ml per minute and, separately collect the four eluates in 500-ml K-D flasks equipped with 10-ml ampuls. Perform the first elution with 200 ml of 6% ethyl ether in petroleum ether, and the second elution with 200 ml of 15% ethyl ether in petro-

leum ether. Perform the third elution with 200 ml of 50% ethyl ether-petroleum ether and the fourth elution with 200 ml of 100% ethyl ether.

10.3.1 Eluate Composition—By using an equivalent quantity of any batch of Florisil as determined by its lauric acid value, the pesticides will be separated into the eluates indicated as follows:

50% Eluate	100% Eluate
Carbaryl (70%)	Carbaryl (30%)
Mexacarbate	Aminocarb
	Propoxur

10.4 Concentrate the eluates to 6–10 ml in the K-D evaporator in a hot water bath. Change to the micro-Snyder column and continue concentration to 0.5–1.0 ml.

10.5 Analyze according to 11, below.

11. Separation and Detection

11.1 Carefully spot 10% of the extract on a thin layer. On the same plate spot several pesticides or mixtures for screening purposes, or a series of 1, 2, 4, 6, 8 and 10 μl of specific standards for quantitative analysis.

11.2 Develop the layers 10 cm in a tank saturated with solvent vapors. Remove the plate and allow it to dry.

11.3 Spray the layer rapidly and evenly with about 10–15 ml chromogenic reagent. Heat the layer in an oven at 110° C for 15 minutes. The pesticides will appear with colors as indicated in Table 2. Make quantitative estimates by visually comparing the intensity and size of the spots with those of the series of standards.

11.4 Spray the layer with sodium borate reagent and observe the color shift of the reaction products. The color shift must be the same for sample and standard for identification to be confirmed.

---

* "Methods for Benzidine, Chlorinated Organic Compounds, Pentachlorophenol and Pesticides in Water and Wastewater" (INTERIM, Pending Issuance of Methods for Organic Analysis of Water and Wastes, September 1978), Environmental Protection Agency, Environmental Monitoring and Support Laboratory (EMSL).

† Also given as Appendix to Section 509A, p. 501, *Standard Methods*, 15th edition.

12. Calculation of Results

12.1 Determine the concentration of pesticide in a sample by comparing the response in a sample to that of a quantity of standard treated on the same layer. Divide the result, in micrograms, by the fraction of extract spotted to convert to micrograms per liter.

13. Reporting Results

13.1 Report results in micrograms per liter without correction for recovery data. When duplicate and spiked samples are analyzed all data obtained should be reported.

Method for N-Aryl Carbamate and Urea Pesticides in Water and Wastewater*

1. Scope and Application

1.1 This method covers the determination of various N-aryl carbamate and urea pesticides in water and wastewater.

1.2 The following pesticides may be determined individually by this method:

Barban
Chlorpropham
Diuron
Fenuron
Fenuron-TCA
Linuron
Monuron
Monuron-TCA
Neburon
Propham
Siduron
Swep

2. Summary

2.1 A measured volume of water is extracted with methylene chloride and the

---

* "Methods for Benzidine, Chlorinated Organic Compounds, Pentachlorophenol and Pesticides in Water and Wastewater" (INTERIM, Pending Issuance of Methods for Organic Analysis of Water and Wastes, September 1978), Environmental Protection Agency, Environmental Monitoring and Support Laboratory (EMSL).

concentrated extract is cleaned up with a Florisil column. Appropriate fractions from the column are concentrated and portions are separated by thin-layer chromatography. The pesticides are hydrolyzed to primary amines, which in turn are chemically converted to diazonium salts. The layer is sprayed with 1-naphthol and the products appear as colored spots. Quantitative measurement is achieved by visually comparing the responses of sample extracts to the responses of standards on the same thin layer. Results are reported in micrograms per liter.

2.2 This method is recommended for use only by experienced pesticide analysts or under the close supervision of such qualified persons.

3. Interferences

3.1 Direct interferences may be encountered from aromatic amines that may be present in the sample. These materials react with the chromogenic reagent and yield reaction products similar to those of the pesticides. In cases where amines are suspected of interfering with a determination, a different solvent system should be used to attempt to isolate the pesticides on the layer.

3.2 Indirect interferences may be encountered from naturally colored materials whose presence masks the chromogenic reaction.

4. Apparatus and Materials

4.1 Thin-layer plates—Glass plates (200 × 200 mm) coated with 0.25 mm layer of Silica Gel G (gypsum binder).

4.2 Spotting Template

4.3 Developing Chamber

4.4 Sprayer—20 ml capacity

4.5 Kuderna-Danish (K-D) Glassware (Kontes)

4.5.1 Snyder Column—three ball (K-503000)

4.5.2 Micro-Snyder Column—two ball (K-569001)

4.5.3 Evaporative Flasks—500 ml (K-57001)

4.5.4 Receiver Ampuls—10 ml graduated (K-570050)

4.5.5 Ampul Stoppers

4.6 Chromatographic Column—Chromaflex (400 mm long × 19 mm ID) with coarse fritted plate on bottom and Teflon stopcock; 250 ml reservoir bulb at top of column with flared out funnel shape at top of bulb—a special order (Kontes K-420540-9011).

4.7 Chromatographic Column—Pyrex (approximately 400 mm long × 20 mm ID) with coarse fritted plate on bottom.

4.8 Micro Syringes—10, 25, 50 and 100 μl.

4.9 Separatory Funnel—2000 ml, with Teflon stopcock.

4.10 Blender—High speed, glass or stainless steel cup.

4.11 Florisil—PR Grade (60–80 mesh); purchase activated at 1250° F and store in the dark in glass containers with glass stoppers or foil-lined screw caps. Before use activate each batch overnight at 130° C in foil-covered glass container. Determine lauric acid value (see Appendix II* †).

5. Reagents, Solvents, and Standards

5.1 Sodium Chloride—(ACS) Saturated solution in distilled water (pre-rinse NaCl with hexane).

5.2 Sodium Hydroxide—(ACS) 10 N in distilled water.

5.3 Sodium Sulfate—(ACS) Granular, anhydrous (conditioned at 400° C for 4 hrs.).

5.4 Sulfuric Acid—(ACS) Mix equal volumes of conc. H_2SO_4 with distilled water.

5.5 Diethyl Ether—Nanograde, redistilled in glass, if necessary.

5.5.1 Must be free of peroxides as indicated by EM Quant test strips. (Test strips are available from EM Laboratories, Inc., 500 Executive Blvd., Elmsford, N.Y. 10523).

5.5.2 Procedures recommended for removal of peroxides are provided with the test strips.

5.6 Hexane, Methanol, Methylene Chloride, Petroleum Ether—nanograde, redistill in glass if necessary.

5.7 Pesticide Standards—Reference grade.

5.7.1 TLC Standards—0.100 μg/μl in chloroform.

5.8 Nitrous acid—prepare just before use by mixing 1 g $NaNO_2$ with 20 ml 0.2 N HCl.

5.9 Chromogenic agent—dissolve 1.0 g l-Naphthol in 20 ml ethanol. Prepare fresh daily.

---

* "Methods for Benzidine, Chlorinated Organic Compounds, Pentachlorophenol and Pesticides in Water and Wastewater" (INTERIM, Pending Issuance of Methods for Organic Analysis of Water and Wastes, September 1978), Environmental Protection Agency, Environmental Monitoring and Support Laboratory (EMSL).

† Also given as Appendix to Section 509A, p. 501, *Standard Methods*, 15th edition.

TABLE 1. R$_f$ VALUES OF N-ARYL CARBAMATE AND UREA PESTICIDES IN SEVERAL SOLVENT SYSTEMS

	A	B	C	D	E	F	G
Carbamates							
Propham	0.49	0.54	0.73	0.48	0.36	0.68	0.69
Chloropropham	0.57	0.60	0.73	0.49	0.37	0.70	0.73
Barban	0.61	0.59	0.72	0.41	0.28	0.70	0.74
Swep	0.48	0.44	0.70	0.41	0.28	0.67	0.66
Urea							
Fenuron	0.03	0.04	0.38	0.22	0.10	0.41	0.30
Fenuron-TCA	0.03	0.04	0.36	0.22	0.10	0.41	0.30
Monuron	0.04	0.05	0.37	0.24	0.10	0.47	0.34
Monuron-TCA	0.04	0.06	0.34	0.24	0.10	0.46	0.34
Diuron	0.05	0.09	0.38	0.28	0.13	0.54	0.44
Linuron	0.40	0.43	0.62	0.39	0.24	0.66	0.64
Neburon	0.21	0.28	0.64	0.41	0.26	0.68	0.65
Siduron	0.02	0.07	0.68	0.39	0.25	0.62	0.55

Solvent Systems: A. Methylene chloride; B. Chloroform; C. Ethyl Acetate; D. Hexane/acetone (2:1); E. Hexane/acetone (4:1); F. Chloroform/acetonitrile (2:1); G. Chloroform/acetonitrile (5:1).

6. Calibration

6.1 To insure even solvent travel up the layer, the tank used for layer development must be thoroughly saturated with developing solvent before it is used. This may be achieved by lining the inner walls of the tank with chromatography paper and introducing the solvent 1–2 hours before use.

6.2 Samples and standards should be introduced to the layer using a syringe, micropipet or other suitable device that permits all the spots to be about the same size and as small as possible. An air stream directed on the layer during spotting will speed solvent evaporation and help to maintain small spots.

6.3 For qualitative and quantitative work, spot a series representing 0.1–1.0 μg of a pesticide. Tables 1 and 2 present color responses and R$_f$ values for several solvent systems.

7. Quality Control

7.1 Duplicate and spiked sample analyses are recommended as quality control checks. Quality control charts (1) should be developed and used as a check on the analytical system. Quality control check samples and performance evaluation samples should be analyzed on a regular basis.

7.2 Each time a set of samples is extracted, a method blank is determined on a volume of distilled water equivalent to that used to dilute the sample.

8. Sample Preparation

8.1 Blend the sample if suspended matter is present and adjust pH to near neutral (pH 6.5–7.5) with 50% sulfuric acid or 10 N sodium hydroxide.

8.2 Quantitatively transfer a one-liter aliquot into a two-liter separatory funnel.

9. Extraction

9.1 Add 60 ml of methylene chloride to the sample in the separatory funnel and shake vigorously for two minutes.

9.2 Allow the solvent to separate from the sample, draw the organic layer into a 100-ml beaker, then pass the organic layer through a chromatographic column containing 3–4 inches anhydrous sodium sulfate, and collect it in a 500-ml K-D flask equipped with a 10-ml ampul. Add a second 60-ml volume of solvent to the separatory funnel and complete the extraction procedure a second time. Perform a third extraction in the same manner.

9.3 Concentrate the extract to 10 ml in a K-D evaporator on a hot water bath. Disconnect the Snyder column just long enough to add 10-ml hexane to the K-D flask and then continue the concentration to about 5–6 ml. If the need for cleanup is indicated, continue to Florisil Column Cleanup (10 below).

9.4 If further cleanup is not required, replace the Snyder column and flask with a micro-Snyder column and continue the concentration to 0.5–1.0 ml. Analyze this final concentrate by thin-layer chromatography (Section 11).

10. Florisil Column Cleanup

10.1 Adjust the sample extract to 10 ml with hexane.

10.2 Place a charge of activated Florisil (weight determined by lauric acid value, see Appendix II* †) in a Chromaflex column. After settling the Florisil by tapping the column, add about one-half inch layer of anhydrous granular sodium sulfate to the top.

10.3 Pre-elute the column, after cooling, with 50–60 ml of petroleum ether. Discard the eluate and just prior to exposure of the sulfate layer to air, quantitatively transfer the sample extract into the column by decantation and subsequent petroleum

* "Methods for Benzidine, Chlorinated Organic Compounds, Pentachlorophenol and Pesticides in Water and Wastewater" (INTERIM, Pending Issuance of Methods for Organic Analysis of Water and Wastes, September 1978), Environmental Protection Agency, Environmental Monitoring and Support Laboratory (EMSL).

† Also given as Appendix to Section 509A, p. 501, *Standard Methods*, 15th edition.

TABLE 2. COLOR RESPONSES AND DETECTION LIMIT FOR THE N-ARYL CARBAMATES AND UREAS

	Color	Detection Limit (ug)
Carbamates		
Propham	Red-purple	0.2
Chloropropham	Purple	0.1
Barban	Purple	0.05
Swep	Blue-purple	0.2
Ureas		
Fenuron	Red-purple	0.05
Fenuron-TCA	Red-purple	0.1
Monuron	Pink-orange	0.05
Monuron-TCA	Pink-orange	0.1
Diuron	Blue-purple	0.1
Linuron	Blue-purple	0.1
Neburon	Blue-purple	0.1
Siduron	Red-purple	0.05

ether washings. Adjust the elution rate to about 5 ml per minute and, separately, collect up to four eluates in 500-ml K-D flasks equipped with 10-ml ampuls. (See Eluate Composition, 10.3.1.) Perform the first elution with 200 ml of 6% ethyl ether in petroleum ether, and the second elution with 200 ml of 15% ethyl ether in petroleum ether. Perform the third elution with 200 ml of 50% ethyl ether-petroleum ether and the fourth elution with 200 ml of 100% ethyl ether.

10.3.1 Eluate Composition—By using an equivalent quantity of any batch of Florisil as determined by its lauric acid value, the pesticides will be separated into the eluates indicated below:

15% Eluate	50% Eluate	100% Eluate
Chlorpropham	Barban (5%)	Neburon (92%)
Propham	Linuron	Diuron
Barban (95%)	Neburon (8%)	Monuron
		Siduron

CAUTION: Fenuron and Fenuron-TCA are not recovered from the Florisil column.

10.4 Concentrate the eluates to 6–10 ml in the K-D evaporator in a hot water bath. Change to the micro-Snyder column and continue concentration to 0.5–1.0 ml.

10.5 Analyze according to 11, below.

11. Separation and Detection

11.1 Carefully spot 10% of the extract on a thin layer. On the same plate spot several pesticides or mixtures for screening purposes, or a series of 1, 2, 4, 6, 8 and 10 μl of specific standards for quantitative analysis.

11.2 Develop the layers 10 cm in a tank saturated with solvent vapors. Remove the plate and allow it to dry.

11.3 Spray the layer rapidly and evenly with about 10–15 ml sulfuric acid solution. Heat the layer in an oven at 110° C for 15 minutes.

11.4 When the layer is cool, spray it with nitrous acid reagent and allow it to dry. Spray the layer with l-naphthol reagent and allow it to dry again. The pesticides will appear as purple spots (see Table 2). Identifications are made by comparison of colors and R_f values. Quantitative estimates are made by visually comparing the intensity and size of the spots with those of the series of standards.

12. Calculation of Results

12.1 Determine the concentration of pesticide in a sample by comparing the response in a sample to that of a quantity of standard treated on the same layer. Divide the result, in micrograms, by the fraction of extract spotted to convert to micrograms per liter.

13. Reporting Results

13.1 Report results in micrograms per liter without correction for recovery data. When duplicate and spiked samples are analyzed all data obtained should be reported.

References

1. "Handbook for Analytical Quality Control in Water and Wastewater Laboratories", Chapter 6, Section 6.4, U. S. Environmental Protection Agency, National Environmental Research Center, Cincinnati, Ohio, 45268, 1972.

Method for Triazine Pesticides in Water and Wastewater*

1. Scope and Application

1.1 This method covers the determination of various symmetrical triazine pesticides in water and wastewaters.

_____

* "Methods for Benzidine, Chlorinated Organic Compounds, Pentachlorophenol and Pesticides in Water and Wastewater" (INTERIM, Pending Issuance of Methods for Organic Analysis of Water and Wastes, September 1978), Environmental Protection Agency, Environmental Monitoring and Support Laboratory (EMSL).

1.2 The following pesticides may be determined individually by this method:

Ametryne
Altraton
Atrazine
Prometon
Prometryn
Propazine
Secbumeton
Simazine
Terbuthylazine

2. Summary

2.1 The method describes an efficient sample extraction procedure and provides, through use of column chromatography, a method for the elimination of non-pesticide interferences and the preseparation of pesticide mixtures. Identification is made by selective gas chromatographic separation, and measurement is accomplished by the use of an electrolytic conductivity detector (CCD) in the nitrogen mode or a nitrogen specific thermionic detector. Results are reported in micrograms per liter.

2.2 This method is recommended for use only by experienced pesticide analysts or under the close supervision of such qualified persons.

3. Interferences

3.1 Solvents, reagents, glassware, and other sample processing hardware may yield discrete artifacts and/or elevated baselines causing misinterpretation of gas chromatograms. All of these materials must be demonstrated to be free from interferences under the conditions of the analysis. Specific selection of reagents and purification of solvents by distillation in all-glass systems may be required. Refer to Appendix I*.

3.2 The interferences in industrial effluents are high and varied and often pose great difficulty in obtaining accurate and precise measurement of triazine pesticides. The use of a specific detector supported by an optional column cleanup procedure will eliminate many of these interferences.

* "Methods for Benzidine, Chlorinated Organic Compounds, Pentachlorophenol and Pesticides in Water and Wastewater" (INTERIM, Pending Issuance of Methods for Organic Analysis of Water and Wastes, September 1978), Environmental Protection Agency, Environmental Monitoring and Support Laboratory (EMSL).

3.3 Nitrogen containing compounds other than the triazines may interfere.

4. Apparatus and Materials

4.1 Gas Chromatograph—Equipped with glass lined injection port.

4.2 Detector Options

4.2.1 Electrolytic Conductivity

4.2.2 Nitrogen specific thermionic

4.3 Recorder—Potentiometric strip chart (10 in.) compatible with the detector.

4.4 Gas Chromatographic Column Materials:

4.4.1 Tubing—Pyrex (180 cm long × 4 mm ID)

4.4.2 Glass Wool—Silanized

4.4.3 Solid Support—Gas Chrom Q (100–120 mesh)

4.4.4 Liquid Phases—Expressed as weight percent coated on solid support.

4.4.4.1 Carbowax 20M, 1%

4.5 Kuderna-Danish (K-D) Glassware

4.5.1 Snyder Column—three ball (macro) and two ball (micro)

4.5.2 Evaporative Flasks—500 ml

4.5.3 Receiver Ampuls—10 ml, graduated

4.5.4 Ampul Stoppers

4.6 Chromatographic Column—Chromaflex (400 mm × 19 mm ID) with coarse fritted plate and Teflon stopcock on bottom; 250 ml reservoir bulb at top of column with flared out funnel shape at top of bulb—a special order (Kontes K-420540-9011).

4.7 Chromatographic Column—Pyrex (approximately 400 mm long × 20 mm ID) with coarse fritted plate on bottom.

4.8 Micro Syringes—10, 25, 50 and 100 μl.

4.9 Separatory funnels—2000 ml with Teflon stopcock.

4.10 Blender—High speed, glass or stainless steel cup.

4.11 Graduated Cylinders—1000 ml.

4.12 Florisil—PR Grade (60–100

mesh); purchase activated at 1250° F and store in the dark in glass containers with glass stoppers or foil-lined screw caps. Before use, activate each batch overnight at 130° C in foil-covered glass container. Determine lauric acid value (See Appendix II* †).

5. Reagents, Solvents, and Standards

5.1 Sodium Hydroxide—(ACS) 10 N in distilled water.

5.2 Sodium Sulfate—(ACS) Granular, anhydrous (conditioned at 400 C for 4 hrs.).

5.3 Sulfuric Acid—(ACS) Mix equal volumes of conc. H_2SO_4 with distilled water.

5.4 Diethyl Ether—Pesticide Quality, redistilled in glass, if necessary.

5.4.1 Must be free of peroxides as indicated by EM Quant Test strips. (Test strips are available from EM Laboratories, Inc., 500 Executive Blvd., Elmsford, N.Y. 10523.)

5.4.2 Procedures recommended for removal of peroxides are provided with the test strips.

5.5 Hexane, Methanol, Methylene Chloride, Petroleum Ether (boiling range 30–60° C)—pesticide quality, redistill in glass if necessary.

5.6 Pesticide Standards—Reference grade.

6. Calibration

6.1 Gas chromatographic operating conditions are considered optimum when

an injection of >20 ng of each triazine will yield a peak at least 50% of full scale deflection with the modified Coulson detector (1). For all quantitative measurements, the detector must be operated within its linear response range and the detector noise level should be less than 2% of full scale.

6.2 Inject standards frequently as a check on the stability of operating conditions. A chromatogram of a mixture of several pesticides is shown in Figure 1 and provides reference operating conditions for the recommended column.

6.3 The elution order and retention ratios of various organophosphorus pesticides are provided in Table 1, as a guide.

7. Quality Control

7.1 Duplicate and spiked sample analyses are recommended as quality control

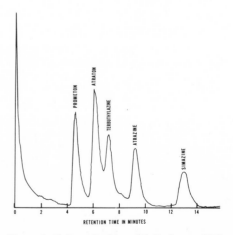

Figure 1. Column Packing: 1% Carbowax 20M on Gas-Chrom Q (100/120 mesh), Column Temperature: 155 C, Carrier Gas: Helium at 80 ml/min, Detector: Electrolytic Conductivity.

---

* "Methods for Benzidine, Chlorinated Organic Compounds, Pentachlorophenol and Pesticides in Water and Wastewater" (INTERIM, Pending Issuance of Methods for Organic Analysis of Water and Wastes, September 1978), Environmental Protection Agency, Environmental Monitoring and Support Laboratory (EMSL).

† Also given as Appendix to Section 509A, p. 501, *Standard Methods*, 15th edition.

TABLE 1. RETENTION RATIOS OF VARIOUS
TRIAZINE PESTICIDES RELATIVE TO ATRAZINE

Pesticide	Retention Ratio
Prometon	0.52
Atraton	0.67
Propazine	0.71
Terbuthylazine	0.78
Secbumeton	0.88
Atrazine	1.00
Prometryne	1.10
Simazine	1.35
Ametryne	1.48

Absolute retention time of atrazine = 10.1 minutes.

checks. Quality control charts (2) should be developed and used as a check on the analytical system. Quality control check samples and performance evaluation samples should be analyzed on a regular basis.

7.2 Each time a set of samples is extracted, a method blank is determined on a volume of distilled water equivalent to that used to dilute the sample.

8. Sample Preparation

8.1 Blend the sample if suspended matter is present and adjust pH to near neutral (pH 6.5–7.5) with 50% sulfuric acid or 10N sodium hydroxide.

8.2 Quantitatively transfer a 1000 ml aliquot into a two-liter separatory funnel.

9. Extraction

9.1 Add 60 ml methylene chloride to the sample in the separatory funnel and shake vigorously for two minutes.

9.2 Allow the solvent to separate from the sample, draw the organic layer into a 100-ml beaker, then pass the organic layer through a chromatographic column containing 3–4 inches anhydrous sodium sulfate, and collect it in a 500-ml K-D flask

equipped with a 10 ml ampul. Add a second 60-ml volume of solvent to the separatory funnel and complete the extraction procedure a second time. Perform a third extraction in the same manner.

9.3 Concentrate the extract to 10 ml in a K-D evaporator on a hot water bath. Disconnect the Snyder column just long enough to add 10 ml hexane to the K-D flask and then continue the concentration to about 5–6 ml. This operation is to displace methylene chloride and give a final hexane solution. If the need for cleanup is indicated, continue to Florisil Column Cleanup (10 below).

9.4 If further cleanup is not required, replace the Snyder column and flask with a micro-Snyder column and continue the concentration to 0.5–1.0 ml. Analyze this final concentrate by gas chromatography.

10. Florisil Column Adsorption Chromatography

10.1 Adjust the sample extract volume to 10 ml.

10.2 Place a charge of activated Florisil (weight determined by lauric acid value, see Appendix II* †) in a Chromaflex column. After settling the Florisil by tapping the column, add about one-half inch layer of anhydrous granular sodium sulfate to the top.

10.3 Pre-elute the column, after cooling, with 50–60 ml of petroleum ether. Discard the eluate and just prior to exposure of the sulfate layer to air, quantitatively transfer the sample extract into the column

---

* "Methods for Benzidine, Chlorinated Organic Compounds, Pentachlorophenol and Pesticides in Water and Wastewater" (INTERIM, Pending Issuance of Methods for Organic Analysis of Water and Wastes, September 1978), Environmental Protection Agency, Environmental Monitoring and Support Laboratory (EMSL).

† Also given as Appendix to Section 509A, p. 501, *Standard Methods,* 15th edition.

by decantation and subsequent petroleum ether washings. Adjust the elution rate to about 5 ml per minute and, separately, collect up to four eluates in 500-ml K-D flasks equipped with 10-ml ampuls. (See Eluate Composition, 10.4.) Perform the first elution with 200 ml of 6% ethyl ether in petroleum ether, and the second elution with 200 ml of 15% ethyl ether in petroleum ether. Perform the third elution with 200 ml of 50% ethyl ether-petroleum ether and the fourth elution with 200 ml of 100% ethyl ether.

10.4 Eluate Composition — By using an equivalent quantity of any batch of Florisil as determined by its lauric acid value, the pesticides will be separated into the eluates indicated as follows:

| | | 100% |
15% Eluate	50% Eluate	Eluate
Propazine (90%)	Propazine (10%)	Atraton
Terbuthyl- azine (30%)	Terbuthyl- azine (70%)	Secbumeton
Atrazine (20%)	Atrazine (80%)	Prometon
	Ametryne	
	Prometryne	
	Simazine	

10.5 Concentrate the eluates to 6–10 ml in the K-D evaporator in a hot water bath. Change to the micro-Snyder column and continue concentration to 0.5–1.0 ml.

10.6 Analyze by gas chromatography.

11. Calculation of Results

11.1 Determine the pesticide concentration by using the absolute calibration procedure described below or the relative calibration procedure described in Appendix III* ‡.

(1) $\text{Micrograms/liter} = \dfrac{(A)(B)(V_t)}{(V_i)(V_s)}$

$A = \dfrac{\text{ng standard}}{\text{standard area}}$

B = Sample aliquot area

V_i = Volume of extract injected (μl)

V_t = Volume of total extract (μl)

V_s = Volume of water extracted (ml)

12. Reporting Results

12.1 Report results in micrograms per liter without correction for recovery data. When duplicate and spiked samples are analyzed all data obtained should be reported.

References

1. Patchett, G. G., "Evaluation of the Electrolytic Conductivity Detector for Residue Analyses of Nitrogen-Containing Pesticides", *Journal of Chromatographic Science*, 8, 155 (1970).
2. "Handbook for Analytical Quality Control in Water and Wastewater Laboratories", Chapter 6, Section 6.4, U. S. Environmental Protection Agency, National Environmental Research Center, Analytical Quality Control Laboratory, Cincinnati, Ohio, 45268, 1972. (Revised edition to be available soon.)

* "Methods for Benzidine, Chlorinated Organic Compounds, Pentachlorophenol and Pesticides in Water and Wastewater" (INTERIM, Pending Issuance of Methods for Organic Analysis of Water and Wastes, September 1978), Environmental Protection Agency, Environmental Monitoring and Support Laboratory (EMSL).

‡ Reproduced following method for Organophosphorus Pesticides, p. S 58.

Insecticides in Water
(Gas Chromatographic Method)*

1. Summary of method

The insecticides are extracted directly from the water sample with n-hexane. After drying and removing the bulk of the solvent, the insecticides are isolated from extraneous material by microcolumn adsorption chromatography. The insecticides are then analyzed by gas chromatography. This method is a modification and extension of the procedures developed by Lamar, Goerlitz, and Law (1965, 1966). For the analysis of insecticides in waters that are grossly polluted by organic compounds other than pesticides, the analyst is referred to the high-capacity cleanup procedure detailed in Federal Water Pollution Control Administration "Method for Chlorinated Hydrocarbon Pesticides in Water and Wastewater" (1969).

2. Application

This method is usable for the analysis of water only. The insecticides and associated chemicals (aldrin, p,p', DDD, p,p'-DDE, o,p'-DDT, p,p'-DDT, dieldrin, endrin, heptachlor, heptachlor epoxide, isodrin, lindane (BHC), and methoxychlor) may be determined to 0.005 μg/l in 1-liter water samples. The insecticides carbophenothion, chlordan, dioxathion, diazinon, ethion, malathion, methyl parathion, Methyl Trithion, parathion, toxaphene, and VC–13 may be determined when present to higher levels (method for organophosphorus pesticides similar to that of Zweig and Devine, 1969). Also, the chemicals chlordene, hexachlorobicycloheptadiene, and hexachlorocyclopenta-

diene, which are pesticide manufacturing precursors, may be analyzed by this method.

3. Interferences

Any compound or compounds having chemical and physical properties similar to the pesticide of interest may cause interference. The procedure incorporates a column chromatographic technique which eliminates most extraneous material. Special precautions are necessary to avoid contamination during sampling and analysis.

4. Apparatus

See step 4, "Gas Chromatographic Analysis of Pesticides."†

4.1 *Concentrating apparatus:* A Kuderna-Danish concentrator, 250-ml capacity with a 1-ball Snyder column, is used for the initial concentration step. Final concentration is performed in the receiver using a 1-ball Snyder microcolumn. A calibrated 4.00-ml receiver tube is used with the concentration apparatus.

4.2 *Cleanup microcolumns:* Disposable Pasteur pipets, 14-cm long and 5-mm ID, are used for the chromatographic cleanup columns. The pipets are washed in warm detergent solution, thoroughly rinsed with dilute hydrochloric acid and organic-free distilled water, then heated to 300°C overnight to remove any traces of organic matter. A column is prepared by plugging the pipet with a small amount of specially cleaned glass wool, adding enough deactivated alumina through a microfunnel to fill 3 cm of the column, followed by another 0.5 cm of anhydrous sodium sulfate.

* "Methods for Analysis of Organic Substances in Water," by D. F. Goerlitz and Eugene Brown, U.S. Geological Survey, Techniques of Water—Resources Investigations, Book 5, Chapter A3 (1972), pp. 30–32.

† Essentially equivalent procedures are given in Method 509A, p. 493, *Standard Methods*, 15th edition.

4.3 *Sandbath,* fluidized, Tecam, or equivalent.

4.4 *Separatory funnels,* Squibb form, 1- or 2-liter capacity. No lubricant is used on the stopcocks.

5. Reagents

5.1 *Alumina,* neutral aluminum oxide, activity grade I, Woelm. Weigh 19 g activated alumina into a 50-ml glass-stoppered erlenmeyer flask and quickly add 1.0 ml distilled water. Stopper the flask and mix the contents thoroughly by tumbling. Allow 2 hr before use. The deactivated alumina may be used for 1 week.

5.2 *Benzene,* distilled in glass, pesticide-analysis quality.

5.3 *n-Hexane,* distilled in glass, pesticide-analysis quality.

5.4 *Sodium sulfate,* anhydrous, granular. Prepare by heating at 300°C overnight and store at 130°C.

5.5 *Water,* distilled, obtained from a high-purity tin-lined still. The feed water is passed through an activated carbon filter. The distillate is collected in a tin-silver-lined storage tank, and the water is constantly irradiated with ultraviolet light during storage. A gravity delivery system is used, and no plastic material other than teflon is allowed to contact the distilled water.

6. Procedure

Samples should be collected according to the recommended practice for the collection of samples for organic analysis. A 1-liter bottle of water should be collected for each sample. No preservative is used. Samples should be shipped promptly. Unless analyzed within a few days, the water should be protected from light and refrigerated. If the sample contains sediment, then the sediment must be analyzed separately. Remove the sediment by centrifugation or filtration through a metal membrane filter. See step 6.1, "Chlorinated Hydrocarbon Insecticides in Suspended Sediment and Bottom Material."‡

All glassware, except volumetric flasks, should be washed in the usual manner, rinsed in dilute hydrochloric acid and distilled water, and heat treated at 300°C overnight. Instead of heat treating, the volumetric ware may be solvent rinsed or steamed to remove organic matter. A reagent and glassware blank should accompany each analysis.

6.1 Water samples (800–900 ml) are extracted with n-hexane in such a manner that the water and the container itself are exposed to the solvent. Weigh the uncapped bottle of water on a triple-beam balance and pour the sample into a 1-liter separatory funnel. Allow the bottle to drain for a few minutes, weigh again, and record the weight of water to three significant figures.

6.2 Add 25 ml n-hexane to the empty sample bottle and gently swirl to wash the sides of the container with the solvent. Pour the contents of the sample bottle into the separatory funnel containing the water. Stopper and shake the separatory funnel vigorously for 1 full min, venting the pressure often. Allow the contents to separate for 10 min and draw off the aqueous layer into the original sample bottle. If the hexane layer emulsifies, separate as much water as possible, then shake the contents of the funnel very vigorously so that the liquids contact the entire inside surface of the vessel. (CAUTION: Vent often!) Allow the layers to separate and add approximately 5 ml distilled water to aid the separation, if necessary. Remove the water and pour the extract from the top of the separatory funnel into a 125-ml erlenmeyer flask containing about 0.5 g anhydrous sodium sulfate.

‡ Reproduced below.

6.3 Repeat a second and third extraction of the water sample in the same manner using 25 ml n-hexane each time, and collect the extracts in the 125-ml erlenmeyer flask containing the drying agent. Cover the flask containing the extract with foil and set aside for 30 min.

6.4 Filter the dried extract through glass wool into the Kuderna-Danish apparatus. Add a sand-sized boiling stone and remove most of the hexane by heating on a fluidized sandbath at 100°C in a hood. When the ball in the Snyder column just stops bouncing, remove the apparatus from the heat and allow to cool. Add another small boiling stone, fit the receiver with a Snyder microcolumn and reduce the volume to between 0.4 and 0.5 ml on the sandbath. Set aside to cool. When changing columns, sand must be cleared from the glass joint before opening.

6.5 Quantitatively transfer the contents of the Kuderna-Danish receiver (0.4–0.5 ml) to the top of a deactivated alumina cleanup microcolumn. Use a disposable pipet to transfer. Not more than 0.1–0.2 ml hexane should be needed for washing. Using hexane, elute the extract from the column to a volume of 8.5 ml in a calibrated 10.00-ml receiver. Add only enough hexane so that the solvent level enters the column packing just as the 8.5-ml elution level is reached. Change receivers and continue the elution using 1:1 benzene-hexane solvent. Collect 8.5 ml of eluate in a second receiver. The first fraction of eluate should contain all the chlorinated hydrocarbon insecticides, and carbophenthion, Methyl Trithion, and VC–13. The remaining phosphorus-containing pesticides are eluted in the benzene-hexane fraction. Reduce the volume of each eluate to 1.00 ml using a Kuderna-Danish microapparatus on the sandbath.

NOTE.—The insecticides are separated chromatographically in a predictable order on the microccolumn, and this may be used to augment gas chromatographic analysis. Although alumina is the adsorbent of choice for the majority of water and sediment samples, occasionally a second pass through a different column is needed for more difficult samples. The analyst is referred to the work of Law and Goerlitz (1970) for a more comprehensive treatment of the cleanup procedure.

6.6 Analyze the eluates by gas chromatography under conditions optimized for the particular gas chromatographic system being used. Run the first analysis on the electron-capture gas chromatograph using the DC–200 column. For components in concentrations ranging from 0.01 μg/l to 1.0 μg/l, a second analysis by electron capture on the QF–1 column is required. Pesticides in concentrations greater than 1.0 μg/l must be analyzed by microcoulometric or flame-photometric gas chromatography on both the DC–200 and the QF–1 columns.

7. Calculations

See step 7, "Gas Chromatographic Analysis."†

8. Report

The pesticide concentrations in water samples are reported as follows: Less than 1.0 μg/l, two decimals and report less than 0.005 μg/l as 0.00 μg/l; 1.0 μg/l and above, to two significant figures. If more than one column or gas chromatographic system is used, report the lowest value.

9. Precision

The results may vary as much as ± 15 percent for compounds in the 0.01- to 0.10-μg/l concentration range. Recovery and precision data are given in table 4.

TABLE 4.—INSECTICIDES IN WATER: RECOVERY OF COMPOUNDS ADDED TO SURFACE-WATER SAMPLES

Insecticide and amount added (μg/l)

Sample No.	Aldrin 0.019	p,p' DDD 0.080	p,p' DDE 0.040	p,p' DDT 0.081	Dieldrin 0.019	Endrin 0.040	Hepta-chlor 0.018	Hepta-chlor epoxide 0.021	Lindane 0.021	Mala-thion 0.181	Methyl para-thion 0.082	Para-thion 0.076
1	82.0	92.5	86.5	95.0	98.8	95.1	86.8	94.0	90.7	92.9	75.1	99.0
2	113	89.1	94.3	97.0	104	98.0	98.7	94.9	101	106	94.6	96.0
3	90.1	96.0	93.5	103	99.6	86.0	95.2	99.2	99.0	120	89.8	110
4	92.1	95.5	92.1	101	104	81.9	96.3	98.1	107	89.3	81.0	86.0
5	97.0	95.0	93.2	96.0	106	81.1	99.6	103	97.5	105	87.8	107
6	89.5	90.5	92.1	96.0	97.7	83.4	95.5	94.2	109	99.3	86.3	84.1
7	91.2	105	95.6	99.0	104	86.6	95.7	99.1	103	107	81.5	103
8	96.1	99.5	96.8	99.0	105	85.0	103	101	115	109	97.1	118
9	95.7	94.0	99.0	102	103	83.3	100	98.3	101	115	91.7	97.9
10	85.0	94.0	98.3	98.0	103	83.3	93.7	98.5	111	103	99.0	101
11	89.9	93.5	95.6	97.5	99.4	90.0	93.3	92.1	99.8	97.8	96.6	85.7
12	86.5	93.0	89.2	92.6	94.9	83.3	90.0	91.7	94.5	101	83.4	87.8
13	91.9	87.6	87.4	93.6	99.3	89.9	99.2	95.4	94.4	106	86.8	124
14	95.3	89.6	90.7	93.1	105	88.2	97.8	100	98.5	89.0	95.1	86.7
15	85.9	86.6	92.8	93.1	104	89.0	88.1	93.4	108	99.6	86.8	88.4
16	96.4	85.6	92.1	88.6	102	90.6	98.1	97.6	102	105	93.7	89.4
17	96.4	84.1	86.5	92.6	104	92.4	99.8	100	101	100	92.1	95.6
18	84.2	98.5	107	104	110	82.5	88.5	90.6	117	107	121	110
Mean	92.1	92.8	93.4	96.7	102	87.2	95.5	96.7	103	103	91	98.3
Variance	49.3	27.9	24.9	17.1	12.9	23.0	21.5	12.5	51.1	63.4	96.5	139.7
Std. dev	7.02	5.28	4.99	4.14	3.59	4.80	4.64	3.54	7.15	7.96	9.82	11.8
Mean error	−7.9	−7.2	−6.6	−3.3	+2.0	−13	−4.5	−3.3	+3.0	+3.0	−9.0	−1.7
Total error[1]	22	18	13	12	9.2	22	14	10	17	19	29	25

[1]McFarren, E. F., Liska, R. J., and Parker, J. H., 1970, Criterion for judging the acceptability of analytical methods: Anal. Chemistry, v. 42, p. 355–358.

References

LAMAR, W. L., GOERLITZ, D. F., and LAW, L. M., 1965, Identification and measurement of chlorinated organic pesticides in water by electron-capture gas chromatography: U.S. Geol. Survey Water-Supply Paper 1817–B, 12 p.

LAMAR, W. L., GOERLITZ, D. F., and LAW, L. M., 1966, Determination of organic insecticides in water by electron-capture gas chromatography, *in* Organic pesticides in the environment: Am. Chem. Soc., Advances in Chemistry, ser. 60, p. 187–199.

LAW, L. M., and GOERLITZ, D. F., 1970, Microcolumn chromatographic cleanup for the analysis of pesticides in water: Assoc. Official Anal. Chemists Jour., v. 53, no. 6, p. 1276–1286.

[U.S.] Federal Water Pollution Control Administration, 1969, FWPCA method for chlorinated hydrocarbon pesticides in water and wastewater: Cincinnati, Federal Water Pollution Control Adm., 29 p.

ZWEIG, GUNTER, and DEVINE, J. M., 1969, Determination of organophosphorus pesticides in water: Residue Rev., v. 26, p. 17–36.

6.1 *Procedure for water samples having suspended sediment*. A reagent blank must accompany the analysis.

6.1.1 Allow the water-sediment sample to remain undisturbed until the sediment has settled. Weigh the uncapped bottles on a balance to three significant figures and carefully decant the water into a separatory funnel of appropriate size. (Separate by centrifugation as in 6.2.2 below and (or) filtration through metal membrane filters if necessary.)

6.1.2 Measure 10 ml acetone or a volume approximately half the equivalent volume of solid, whichever is greater, into the sample bottle containing the sediment. Replace the cap and gently mix the contents of the bottle on a shaker table for 20 min. Add 25 ml n-hexane and mix the contents for an additional 10 min. Decant the extract into the separatory funnel containing the water from the sample. Repeat the extraction of the sediment in the same manner two more times, using fresh acetone and hexane each time.

NOTE.—Additional hexane may be needed to recover the acetone extract from the sediment. Also, the extract may have to be filtered through a plug of glass wool. Anhydrous sodium sulfate may be added to aid in separating the solvent from the sediment. Add the sodium sulfate slowly and mix to the desired consistency. A quantity of sodium sulfate equal to the amount of sediment may be added if necessary.

6.1.3 Shake the combined extracts with the water from the sample for 1 min. Rinse the sediment from the sample bottle with distilled water and collect the water from the sample in the sample bottle. The sediment may be discarded. Decant the extract from the top of the separatory funnel into a 250-ml erlenmeyer flask.

6.1.4 Extract the water from the sample with an additional 25 ml hexane and discard the water. Weigh the sample bottle to determine the weight of the sample.

6.1.5 Combine the extracts in the separatory funnel and wash two times with 500 ml distilled water each time. Collect the extract in the 250-ml erlenmeyer flask containing approximately 0.5 g Na_2SO_4, and continue the analysis as in the procedure, beginning step 6.4, "Insecticides in Water."

Method for Polychlorinated Biphenyls (PCBs) in Water and Wastewater*

1. Scope and Application

1.1 This method covers the determination of various polychlorinated biphenyl (PCB) mixtures in water and wastewater.

1.2 The following mixtures of chlorinated biphenyls (Aroclors) may be determined by this method:

PCB-1016
PCB-1221
PCB-1232
PCB-1242
PCB-1248
PCB-1254
PCB-1260

1.3 The method is an extension of the Method for Chlorinated Hydrocarbons in Water and Wastewater (1). It is designed so that determination of both the PCBs and the organochlorine pesticides may be made on the same sample.

2. Summary

2.1 The PCBs and the organochlorine pesticides are co-extracted by liquid-liquid extraction and, insofar as possible, the two classes of compounds separated from one another prior to gas chromatographic determination. A combination of the standard Florisil column cleanup procedure and a silica gel microcolumn separation procedure (2)(3) are employed. Identification is made from gas chromatographic patterns obtained through the use of two or more unlike columns. Detection and measurement is accomplished using an electron capture, microcoulometric, or electrolytic conductivity detector. Techniques for confirming qualitative identification are suggested.

3. Interferences

3.1 Solvents, reagents, glassware, and other sample processing hardware may yield discrete artifacts and/or elevated baselines causing misinterpretation of gas chromatograms. All of these materials must be demonstrated to be free from interferences under the conditions of the analysis. Specific selection of reagents and the purification of solvents by distillation in all-glass systems may be required. Refer to Appendix I* †.

3.2 The interferences in industrial effluents are high and varied and pose great difficulty in obtaining accurate and precise measurement of PCBs and organochlorine pesticides. Separation and clean-up procedures are generally required and may result in the loss of certain organochlorine compounds. Therefore, great care should be exercised in the selection and use of methods for eliminating or minimizing interferences. It is not possible to describe procedures for overcoming all of the interferences that may be encountered in industrial effluents.

3.3 Phthalate esters, certain organophosphorus pesticides, and elemental sulfur will interfere when using electron capture for detection. These materials do not interfere when the microcoulometric or electrolytic conductivity detectors are used in the halogen mode.

3.4 Organochlorine pesticides and other

---

* "Methods for Benzidine, Chlorinated Organic Compounds, Pentachlorophenol and Pesticides in Water and Wastewater" (INTERIM, Pending Issuance of Methods for Organic Analysis of Water and Wastes, September 1978), Environmental Protection Agency, Environmental Monitoring and Support Laboratory (EMSL).

† Reproduced following method for Organophosphorus Pesticides, p. S 58.

halogenated compounds constitute interferences in the determination of PCBs. Most of these are separated by the method described below. However, certain compounds, if present in the sample, will occur with the PCBs. Included are: Sulfur, Heptachlor, aldrin, DDE, technical chlordane, mirex, and to some extent, o,p'-DDT and p,p'-DDT.

4. Apparatus and Materials

4.1 Gas Chromatograph—Equipped with glass lined injection port.

4.2 Detector Options:

4.2.1 Electron Capture—Radioactive (tritium or nickel-63)

4.2.2 Microcoulometric Titration

4.2.3 Electrolytic Conductivity

4.3 Recorder—Potentiometric strip chart (10 in.) compatible with the detector.

4.4 Gas Chromatographic Column Materials:

4.4.1 Tubing—Pyrex (180 cm long × 4 mm ID)

4.4.2 Glass Wool—Silanized

4.4.3 Solid Support—Gas-Chrom Q (100–120 mesh)

4.4.4 Liquid Phases—Expressed as weight percent coated on solid support.

4.4.4.1 SE-30 or OV-1, 3%

4.4.4.2 OV-17, 1.5% + QF-1 or OV-210, 1.95%

4.5 Kuderna-Danish (K-D) Glassware

4.5.1 Snyder Column—three-ball (macro) and two-ball (micro)

4.5.2 Evaporative Flasks—500 ml

4.5.3 Receiver Ampuls—10 ml, graduated

4.5.4 Ampul Stoppers

4.6 Chromatographic Column—Chromaflex (400 mm long × 19 mm ID) with coarse fritted plate on bottom and Teflon stopcock: 250 ml-reservoir bulb at top of column with flared out funnel shape at top of bulb—a special order (Kontes K-420540-9011).

4.7 Chromatographic Column—pyrex (approximately 400 mm long × 20 mm ID) with coarse fritted plate on bottom.

4.8 Micro Column Pyrex—constructed according to Figure 1.

4.9 Capillary pipets disposable (5-3/4 in.) with rubber bulb (Scientific Products P5205-1).

4.10 Low pressure regulator—0 to 5 PSIG—with low-flow needle valve (see Figure 1, Matheson Model 70).

4.11 Beaker—100 ml

4.12 Micro Syringes—10, 25, 50 and 100 μl.

4.13 Separatory funnels—125 ml, 1000 ml and 2000 ml with Teflon stopcock.

4.14 Blender—High speed, glass or stainless steel cup.

4.15 Graduated cylinders—100 and 250 ml.

4.16 Florisil—PR Grade (60–100 mesh); purchase activated at 1250° F and store in the dark in glass containers with glass stoppers or foil-lined screw caps. Before use, activate each batch overnight at 130° C in foil-covered glass container. Determine lauric-acid value (See Appendix II* ‡.)

4.17 Silica gel—Davison code 950-08008-226 (60/200 mesh).

4.18 Glass Wool—Hexane extracted.

4.19 Centrifuge Tubes—Pyrex calibrated (15 ml).

5. Reagents, Solvents, and Standards

5.1 Sodium Chloride—(ACS) Saturated solution in distilled water (pre-rinse NaCl with hexane).

---

* "Methods for Benzidine, Chlorinated Organic Compounds, Pentachlorophenol and Pesticides in Water and Wastewater" (INTERIM, Pending Issuance of Methods for Organic Analysis of Water and Wastes, September 1978), Environmental Protection Agency, Environmental Monitoring and Support Laboratory (EMSL).

‡ Also given as Appendix to Section 509A, p. 501, *Standard Methods,* 15th edition.

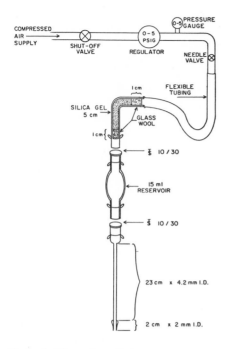

Figure 1. Microcolumn System.

5.2 Sodium Hydroxide—(ACS) 10 N in distilled water.

5.3 Sodium Sulfate—(ACS) Granular, anhydrous (conditioned at 400° C for 4 hrs.).

5.4 Sulfuric Acid—(ACS) Mix equal volumes of conc. H_2SO_4 with distilled water.

5.5 Diethyl Ether—Nanograde, redistilled in glass, if necessary.

5.5.1 Must be free of peroxides as indicated by EM Quant test strips. (Test strips are available from EM Laboratories, Inc., 500 Executive Blvd., Elmsford, N.Y. 10523).

5.5.2 Procedures recommended for removal of peroxides are provided with the test strips.

5.6 n-Hexane—Pesticide quality (NOT MIXED HEXANES).

5.7 Acetonitrile, Hexane, Methanol, Methylene Chloride, Petroleum Ether (boiling range 30–60°C)—pesticide quality, redistill in glass if necessary.

5.8 Standards—Aroclors 1221, 1232, 1242, 1248, 1254, 1260, and 1016.

5.9 Anti-static Solution—STATNUL, Daystrom, Inc., Weston Instrument Division, Newark, N.J., 95212.

6. Calibration

6.1 Gas chromatographic operating conditions are considered acceptable if the response to dicapthon is at least 50% of full scale when ≲ 0.06 ng is injected for electron capture detection and ≲ 100 ng is injected for microcoulometric or electrolytic conductivity detection. For all quantitative measurements, the detector must be operated within its linear response range and the detector noise level should be less than 2% of full scale.

6.2 Standards are injected frequently as a check on the stability of operating conditions, detector and column. Example chromatograms are shown in Figures 3 through 8 and provide reference operating conditions.

7. Quality Control

7.1 Duplicate and spiked sample analyses are recommended as quality control checks. Quality control charts (4) should be developed and used as a check on the analytical system. Quality control check samples and performance evaluation samples should be analyzed on a regular basis.

7.2 Each time a set of samples is extracted, a method blank is determined on a volume of distilled water equivalent to that used to dilute the sample.

8. Sample Preparation

8.1 Blend the sample if suspended matter is present and adjust pH to near neutral (pH 6.5–7.5) with 50% sulfuric acid or 10 N sodium hydroxide.

8.2 For sensitivity requirement of 1 μg/l, when using microcoulometric or electrolytic conductivity methods for detection take 1000 ml of sample for analysis. If interferences pose no problem, the sensitivity of the electron capture detector should permit as little as 100 ml of sample to be used. Background information on the extent and nature of interferences will assist the analyst in choosing the required sample size and preferred detector.

8.3 Quantitatively transfer the proper aliquot into a two-liter separatory funnel and dilute to one liter.

9. Extraction

9.1 Add 60 ml of 15% methylene chloride in hexane (v:v) to the sample in the separatory funnel and shake vigorously for two minutes.

9.2 Allow the mixed solvent to separate from the sample, then draw the water into a one-liter Erlenmeyer flask. Pour the organic layer into a 100-ml beaker and then pass it through a column containing 3–4 inches of anhydrous sodium sulfate, and collect it in a 500-ml K-D flask equipped with a 10 ml-ampul. Return the water phase to the separatory funnel. Rinse the Erlenmeyer flask with a second 60-ml volume of solvent; add the solvent to the separatory funnel and complete the extraction procedure a second time. Perform a third extraction in the same manner.

9.3 Concentrate the extract in the K-D evaporator on a hot water bath.

9.4 Qualitatively analyze the sample by gas chromatography with an electron capture detector. From the response obtained decide:

a. If there are any organochlorine pesticides present.

b. If there are any PCBs present.

c. If there is a combination of a and b.

d. If elemental sulfur is present.

e. If the response is too complex to determine a, b or c.

f. If no response, concentrate to 1.0 ml or less, as required, and repeat the analysis looking for a, b, c, d and e. Samples containing Aroclors with a low percentage of chlorine, e.g., 1221 and 1232, may require this concentration in order to achieve the detection limit of 1 μg/l. Trace quantitites of PCBs are often masked by background which usually occur in samples.

9.5 If condition *a* exists, quantitatively determine the organochlorine pesticides according to (1).

9.6 If condition *b* exists, PCBs only are present: no further separation or cleanup is necessary. Quantitatively determine the PCBs according to step 11.

9.7 If condition *c* exists, compare peaks obtained from the sample to those of standard Aroclors and make a judgment as to which Aroclors may be present. To separate the PCBs from the organochlorine pesticides, continue as outlined in 10.4.

9.8 If condition *d* exists, separate the sulfur from the sample using the method outlined in 10.3 followed by the method in 10.5.

9.9 If condition *e* exists, the following macro cleanup and separation procedures (10.2 and 10.3) should be employed and, if necessary, followed by the micro separation procedures (10.4 and 10.5).

10. Cleanup and Separation Procedures

10.1 Interferences in the form of distinct peaks and/or high background in the initial gas chromatographic analysis, as well as the physical characteristics of the extract (color, cloudiness, viscosity) and background knowledge of the sample will indicate whether clean-up is required. When these interfere with measurement of the PCBs, or affect column life or detector sensitivity, proceed as directed below.

10.2 Acetonitrile Partition—This procedure is used to remove fats and oils from the sample extracts. It should be noted that not all pesticides are quantitatively recovered by this procedure. The analyst must be aware of this and demonstrate the efficiency of the partitioning for the compounds of interest.

10.2.1 Quantitatively transfer the previously concentrated extract to a 125-ml separatory funnel with enough hexane to bring the final volume to 15 ml. Extract the sample four times by shaking vigorously for one minute with 30-ml portions of hexane-saturated acetonitrile.

10.2.2 Combine and transfer the acetonitrile phases to a one-liter separatory funnel and add 650 ml of distilled water and 40 ml of saturated sodium chloride solution. Mix thoroughly for 30–45 seconds. Extract with two 100-ml portions of hexane by vigorously shaking about 15 seconds.

10.2.3 Combine the hexane extracts in a one-liter separatory funnel and wash with two 100-ml portions of distilled water. Discard the water layer and pour the hexane layer through a 3–4 inch anhydrous sodium sulfate column into a 500-ml K-D flask equipped with a 10-ml ampul. Rinse the separatory funnel and column with three 10-ml portions of hexane.

10.2.4 Concentrate the extracts to 6–10 ml in the K-D evaporator in a hot water bath.

10.2.5 Analyze by gas chromatography unless a need for further cleanup is indicated.

10.3 Florisil   Column   Adsorption Chromatography

10.3.1 Adjust   the   sample   extract volume to 10 ml.

10.3.2 Place a charge of activated Florisil (weight   determined   by   lauric-acid

value, see Appendix II* ‡) in a Chromaflex column. After settling the Florisil by tapping the column, add about one-half inch layer of anhydrous granular sodium sulfate to the top.

10.3.3 Pre-elute the column, after cooling, with 50–60 ml of petroleum ether. Discard the eluate and just prior to exposure of the sulfate layer to air, quantitatively transfer the sample extract into the column by decantation and subsequent petroleum ether washings. Adjust the elution rate to about 5 ml per minute and, separately, collect up to three eluates in 500-ml K-D flasks equipped with 10-ml ampuls (see Eluate Composition 10.3.3.1). Perform the first elution with 200 ml of 6% ethyl ether in petroleum ether, and the second elution with 200 ml of 15% ethyl ether in petroleum ether. Perform the third elution with 200 ml of 50% ethyl ether—petroleum ether and the fourth elution with 200 ml of 100% ethyl ether.

10.3.3.1 Eluate Composition—By using an equivalent quantity of any batch of Florisil as determined by its lauric acid value, the pesticides will be separated into the eluates indicated as follows.

6% Eluate		
Aldrin	DDT	Pentachloro-
BHC	Heptachlor	nitrobenzene
Chlordane	Heptachlor	Strobane
DDD	Epoxide	Toxaphene
DDE	Lindane	Trifluralin
	Methoxychlor	PCBs
	Mirex	

---

* "Methods for Benzidine, Chlorinated Organic Compounds, Pentachlorophenol and Pesticides in Water and Wastewater" (INTERIM, Pending Issuance of Methods for Organic Analysis of Water and Wastes, September 1978), Environmental Protection Agency, Environmental Monitoring and Support Laboratory (EMSL).

‡ Also given as Appendix to Section 509A, p. 501, *Standard Methods*, 15th edition.

15% Eluate	50% Eluate
Endosulfan I	Endosulfan II
Endrin	Captan
Dieldrin	
Dichloran	
Phthalate esters	

Certain thiophosphate pesticides will occur in each of the above fractions as well as the 100% fraction. For additional information regarding eluate composition, refer to the FDA Pesticide Analytical Manual (5).

10.3.4 Concentrate the eluates to 6-10 ml in the K-D evaporator in a hot water bath.

10.3.5 Analyze by gas chromatography.

10.4 Silica Gel Micro-Column Separation Procedure (6)

10.4.1 Activation for Silica Gel

10.4.1.1 Place about 20 gm of silica gel in a 100-ml beaker. Activate at 180° C for approximately 16 hours. Transfer the silica gel to a 100-ml glass-stoppered bottle. When cool, cover with about 35 ml of 0.50% diethyl ether in benzene (volume: volume). Keep bottle well sealed. If silica gel collects on the ground glass surfaces, wash off with the above solvent before resealing. Always maintain an excess of the mixed solvent in bottle (approximately 1/2 in. above silica gel). Silica gel can be effectively stored in this manner for several days.

10.4.2 Preparation of the Chromatographic Column

10.4.2.1 Pack the lower 2 mm ID section of the microcolumn with glass wool. Permanently mark the column 120 mm above the glass wool. Using a clean rubber bulb from a disposable pipet seal the lower end of the microcolumn. Fill the microcolumn with 0.50% ether in benzene (v:v) to the bottom of the 10/30 joint (Figure 1). Using a disposable capillary pipet, transfer several aliquots of the silica gel slurry into the microcolumn. After approximately 1 cm of silica gel collects in the bottom of the microcolumn, remove the rubber bulb seal, tap the column to insure that the silica gel reaches the 120 ± 2 mm mark. Be sure that there are no air bubbles in the column. Add about 10 mm of sodium sulfate to the top of the silica gel. Under low humidity conditions, the silica gel may coat the sides of the column and not settle properly. This can be minimized by wiping the outside of the column with an antistatic solution.

10.4.2.2 Deactivation of the Silica Gel

a. Fill the microcolumn to the base of the 10/30 joint with the 0.50% ether-benzene mixture, assemble reservoir (using spring clamps) and fill with approximately 15 ml of the 0.50% ether-benzene mixture. Attach the air pressure device (using spring clamps) and adjust the elution rate to approximately 1 ml/min. with the air pressure control. Release the air pressure and detach reservoir just as the last of the solvent enters the sodium sulfate. Fill the column with n-hexane (not mixed hexanes) to the base of the 10/30 fitting. Evaporate all residual benzene from the reservoir, assemble the reservoir section and fill with 5 ml of n-hexane. Apply air pressure and remove the reservoir just as the n-hexane enters the sodium sulfate. The column is now ready for use.

b. Pipet a 1.0 ml aliquot of the concentrated sample extract (previously reduced to a total volume of 2.0 ml) on to the column. As the last of the sample passes into the sodium sulfate layer, rinse down the internal wall of the column twice with 0.25 ml of n-hexane. Then assemble the upper section of the column. As the last of the n-hexane rinse reaches the surface of the sodium sulfate, add enough n-hexane (volume predetermined, see 10.4.3) to just elute all of the PCBs present in the sample. Apply air pressure and adjust until the flow is 1 ml/min. Collect the desired volume of eluate (predetermined, see 10.4.3) in an accurately calibrated ampul. As the last of the n-hexane reaches the surface of the sodium sulfate, release the air pressure and change the collection ampul.

c. Fill the column with 0.50% diethyl ether in benzene, again apply air pressure and adjust flow to 1 ml/min. Collect the eluate until all of the organochlorine pesticides of interest have been eluted (volume predetermined, see 10.4.3).

d. Analyze the eluates by gas chromatography.

10.4.3 Determination of Elution Volumes

10.4.3.1 The elution volumes for the PCBs and the pesticides depend upon a number of factors which are difficult to control. These include variation in:

a. Mesh size of the silica gel

b. Adsorption properties of the silica gel

c. Polar contaminants present in the eluting solvent

d. Polar materials present in the sample and sample solvent

e. The dimensions of the microcolumns. Therefore, the optimum elution volume must be experimentally determined each time a factor is changed. To determine the elution volumes, add standard mixtures of Aroclors and pesticides to the column and serially collect 1-ml elution volumes. Analyze the individual eluates by gas chromatography and determine the cut-off volume for n-hexane and for ether-benzene. Figure 2 shows the retention order of the various PCB components and of the pesticides. Using this information, prepare the mixtures required for calibration of the microcolumn.

10.4.3.2 In determining the volume of hexane required to elute the PCBs the sample volume (1 ml) and the volume of n-hexane used to rinse the column wall must be considered. Thus, if it is determined that a 10.0-ml elution volume is required to elute the PCBs, the volume of hexane to be added in addition to the sample volume but including the rinse volume should be 9.5 ml.

10.4.3.3 Figure 2 shows that as the average chlorine content of a PCB mixture decreases the solvent volume for complete elution increases. Qualitative determination (9.4) indicates which Aroclors are present and provides the basis for selection of the ideal elution volume. This helps to minimize the quantity of organochlorine pesticides which will elute along with the low percent chlorine PCBs and insures the most efficient separations possible for accurate analysis.

10.4.3.4 For critical analysis where the PCBs and pesticides are not separated completely, the column should be accurately calibrated according to (10.4.3.1) to determine the percent of material of interest that elutes in each fraction. Then flush the column with an additional 15 ml of n-hexane and use this reconditioned column for the sample separation. Using this technique one can accurately predict the amount (%) of materials in each micro column fraction.

10.5 Micro Column Separation of Sulfur, PCBs, and Pesticides

10.5.1 See procedure for preparation and packing micro column in PCB analysis section (10.4.1 and 10.4.2).

10.5.2 Microcolumn Calibration

10.5.2.1 Calibrate the microcolumn for sulfur and PCB separation by collecting 1.0-ml fractions and analyzing them by gas chromatography to determine the following:

1) The fraction with the first eluting PCBs (those present in 1260),

2) The fraction with the last eluting PCBs (those present in 1221),

3) The elution volume for sulfur,

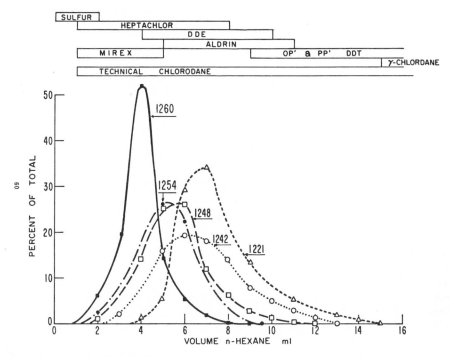

Figure 2. Aroclor Elution Patterns.

4) The elution volume for the pesticides of interest in the 0.50% ether-benzene fraction.

From these data determine the following:

1) The eluting volume containing only sulfur (Fraction I),

2) The eluting volume containing the last of the sulfur and the early eluting PCBs (Fraction II),

3) The eluting volume containing the remaining PCBs (Fraction III),

4) The ether-benzene eluting volume containing the pesticides of interest (Fraction IV).

10.5.3 Separation Procedure

10.5.3.1 Carefully concentrate the 6% eluate from the florisil column to 2.0 ml in the graduated ampul on a warm water bath.

10.5.3.2 Place 1.0 ml (50%) of the concentrate into the microcolumn with a 1-ml pipet. Be careful not to get any sulfur crystals into the pipet.

10.5.3.3 Collect Fractions I and II in calibrated centrifuge tubes. Collect Fractions III and IV in calibrated ground glass stoppered ampuls.

10.5.3.4 Sulfur Removal (7)—Add 1 to 2 drops of mercury to Fraction II stopper and place on a wrist-action shaker. A black precipitate indicates the presence of sulfur. After approximately 20 minutes the mercury may become entirely reacted or deactivated by the precipitate. The sample should be quantitatively transferred to a clean centrifuge tube and additional mercury added. When crystals are present in the sample, three treatments may be necessary to remove all the sulfur. After all the sulfur has been removed from Fraction II (check using gas chromatography) combine Fractions II and III. Adjust the volume to 10 ml and analyze by gas chromatography. Be sure no mercury is transferred to the combined Fractions II and III, since it can react with certain pesticides.

By combining Fractions II and III, if PCBs are present, it is possible to identify the Aroclor(s) present and a quantitative analysis can be performed accordingly. Fraction I can be discarded since it only contains the bulk of the sulfur. Analyze Fractions III and IV for the PCBs and pesticides. If DDT and its homologs, aldrin, heptachlor, or technical chlordane are present along with the PCBs, an additional microcolumn separation can be performed which may help to further separate the PCBs from the pesticides (See 10.4).

11. Quantitative Determination

11.1 Measure the volume of n-hexane eluate containing the PCBs and inject 1 to 5 μl into the gas chromatograph. If necessary, adjust the volume of the eluate to give linear response to the electron capture detector. The microcoulometric or the electrolytic detector may be employed to improve specificity for samples having higher concentrations of PCBs.

11.2 Calculations

11.2.1 When a single Aroclor is present, compare quantitative Aroclor reference standards (e.g., 1242, 1260) to the unknown. Measure and sum the areas of the unknown and the reference Aroclor and calculate the result as follows:

$$\text{Microgram/liter} = \frac{[A]\,[B]\,[V_d]}{[(V_i)\,(V_s)]} \times [N]$$

$A = \dfrac{\text{ng of Standard Injected}}{\text{area}} = \dfrac{\text{ng}}{\text{mm}^2}$

B = Sum of sample peak areas (mm^2)

V_i = Volume of extract (μl) from which sample is injected into gas chromatograph

V_s = Volume of water sample extracted (ml)

N = 2 when micro column used
    1 when micro column not used

Peak area = peak height (mm $\times$ peak width at 1/2 height

11.2.2 For complex situations, use the calibration method described below (8). Small variations in components between different Aroclor batches make it necessary to obtain samples of several specific Aroclors. These reference Aroclors can be obtained from the Southeast Environmental Research Laboratory, EPA, Athens, Georgia, 30601. The procedure is as follows:

11.2.2.1 Using the OV-1 column, chromatograph a known quantity of each Aroclor reference standard. Also chromatograph a sample of p,p'-DDE. Suggested concentration of each standard is 0.1 ng/μl for the Aroclors and 0.02 ng/μl for the p,p'-DDE.

11.2.2.2 Determine the relative retention time (RRT) of each PCB peak in the resulting chromatograms using p,p'-DDE as 100.

$$RRT = \frac{RT \times 100}{RT_{DDE}}$$

RRT = Relative Retention Time
RT = Retention time of peak of interest
RT_{DDE} = Retention time of p,p'-DDE

Retention time is measured as that distance in mm between the first appearance of the solvent peak and the maximum for the compound.

11.2.2.3 To calibrate the instrument for each PCB measure the area of each peak. Area = peak height (mm) $\times$ peak width at 1/2 height. Using Tables 1 through 6 obtain the proper mean weight factor, then determine the response factor ng/mm^2.

$$ng/mm^2 = \frac{(ng_i)\frac{(mean\ weight\ percent)}{100}}{(Area)}$$

ng_i = ng of Aroclor Standard Injected

Mean weight percent—obtained from Tables 1 through 6.

11.2.2.4 Calculate the RRT value and the area for each PCB peak in the sample chromatogram. Compare the sample chromatogram to those obtained for each reference Aroclor standard. If it is apparent that the PCB peaks present are due to only one Aroclor, then calculate the concentration of each PCB using the following formula:

ng PCB = ng/mm^2 × Area

Where Area = Area (mm^2) of sample peak
ng/mm^2 = Response factor for that peak measured.

TABLE 1. COMPOSITION OF AROCLOR 1221 (8)

RRT[a]	Mean Weight Percent	Relative Std. Dev.[b]	Number of Chlorines[c]	
11	31.8	15.8	1	
14	19.3	9.1	1	
16	10.1	9.7	2	
19	2.8	9.7	2	
21	20.8	9.3	2	
28	5.4	13.9	2 3	85% 15%
32	1.4	30.1	2 3	10% 90%
37 40	1.7	48.8	3	

[a] Retention time relative to p,p′-DDE = 100. Measured from first appearance of solvent. Overlapping peaks that are quantitated as one peak are bracketed.
[b] Relative standard deviation of seventeen results.
[c] From GC-MS data. Peaks containing mixtures of isomers of different chlorine numbers are bracketed.

TABLE 2. COMPOSITION OF AROCLOR 1232 (8)

RRT[a]	Mean Weight Percent	Relative Std. Dev.[b]	Number of Chlorines[c]	
11	16.2	3.4	1	
14	9.9	2.5	1	
16	7.1	6.8	2	
20 21	17.8	2.4	2	
28	9.6	3.4	2 3	40% 60%
32	3.9	4.7	3	
37	6.8	2.5	3	
40	6.4	2.7	3	
47	4.2	4.1	4	
54	3.4	3.4	3 4	33% 67%
58	2.6	3.7	4	
70	4.6	3.1	4 5	90% 10%
78	1.7	7.5	4	
Total	94.2			

[a] Retention time relative to p,p′-DDE = 100. Measured from first appearance of solvent. Overlapping peaks that are quantitated as one peak are bracketed.
[b] Relative standard deviation of four results.
[c] From GC-MS data. Peaks containing mixtures of isomers of different chlorine numbers are bracketed.

Then add the nanograms of PCBs present in the injection to get the total number of nanograms of PCBs present. Use the following formula to calculate the concentration of PCBs in the sample:

$$Micrograms/Liter = \frac{ng\ PCBs \times V_t \times N}{V_i \times V_s}$$

V_s = volume of water extracted (ml)
V_t = volume of extract (μl)
V_i = volume of sample injected (μl)
ng = sum of all the PCBs in nanograms for that Aroclor identified
N = 2 when microcolumn used
N = 1 when microcolumn not used

The value can then be reported as

TABLE 3. COMPOSITION OF AROCLOR 1242 (8)

RRT[a]	Mean Weight Percent	Relative Std. Dev.[b]	Number of Chlorines[c]	
11	1.1	35.7	1	
16	2.9	4.2	2	
21	11.3	3.0	2	
28	11.0	5.0	2	25%
			3	75%
32	6.1	4.7	3	
37	11.5	5.7	3	
40	11.1	6.2	3	
47	8.8	4.3	4	
54	6.8	2.9	3	33%
			4	67%
58	5.6	3.3	4	
70	10.3	2.8	4	90%
			5	10%
78	3.6	4.2	4	
84	2.7	9.7	5	
98	1.5	9.4	5	
104	2.3	16.4	5	
125	1.6	20.4	5	85%
			6	15%
146	1.0	19.9	5	75%
			6	25%

[a] Retention time relative to p,p'-DDE = 100. Measured from first appearance of solvent.

[b] Relative standard deviation of six results.

[c] From GC-MS data. Peaks containing mixtures of isomers of different chlorine numbers are bracketed.

TABLE 4. COMPOSITION OF AROCLOR 1248 (8)

RRT[a]	Mean Weight Percent	Relative Std. Dev.[b]	Number of Chlorines[c]	
21	1.2	23.9	2	
28	5.2	3.3	3	
32	3.2	3.8	3	
47	8.3	3.6	3	
40	8.3	3.9	3	85%
			4	15%
47	15.6	1.1	4	
54	9.7	6.0	3	10%
			4	90%
58	9.3	5.8	4	
70	19.0	1.4	4	80%
			5	20%
78	6.6	2.7	4	
84	4.9	2.6	5	
98	3.2	3.2	5	
104	3.3	3.6	4	10%
			5	90%
112	1.2	6.6	5	
125	2.6	5.9	5	90%
			6	10%
146	1.5	10.0	5	85%
			6	15%
Total	103.1			

[a] Retention time relative to p,p'-DDE = 100. Measured from first appearance of solvent.

[b] Relative standard deviation of six results.

[c] From GC-MS data. Peaks containing mixtures of isomers of different chlorine numbers are bracketed.

micrograms/liter PCBs or as the Aroclor. For samples containing more than one Aroclor, use Figure 9 chromatogram divisional flow chart to assign a proper response factor to each peak and also identify the "most likely" Aroclors present. Calculate the ng of each PCB isomer present and sum them according to the divisional flow chart. Using the formula above, calculate the concentration of the various Aroclors present in the sample.

12. Reporting Results

12.1 Report results in micrograms per liter without correction for recovery data.

When duplicate and spiked samples are analyzed, all data obtained should be reported.

References

1. "Method for Chlorinated Hydrocarbons in Water and Wastewater", EPA Interim Methods, Sept. 1978, p. 7.
2. Leoni, V., "The Separation of Fifty Pesticides and Related Compounds and Polychlorinated Biphenyls into Four Groups by Silica Gel Microcolumn Chromatography", *Journal of Chromatography*, 62, 63 (1971).
3. McClure, V. E., "Precisely Deactivated Adsorbents Applied to the Separation of Chlor-

TABLE 5. COMPOSITION OF AROCLOR 1254 (8)

RRT[a]	Mean Weight Percent	Relative Std. Dev.[b]	Number of Chlorines[c]	
47	6.2	3.7	4	
54	2.9	2.6	4	
58	1.4	2.8	4	
70	13.2	2.7	4	25%
			5	75%
84	17.3	1.9	5	
98	7.5	5.3	5	
104	13.6	3.8	5	
125	15.0	2.4	5	70%
			6	30%
146	10.4	2.7	5	30%
			6	70%
160	1.3	8.4	6	
174	8.4	5.5	6	
203	1.8	18.6	6	
232	1.0	26.1	7	
Total	100.0			

[a] Retention time relative to p,p′-DDE = 100. Measured from first appearance of solvent.

[b] Relative standard deviation of six results.

[c] From GC-MS data. Peaks containing mixtures of isomers are bracketed.

TABLE 6. COMPOSITION OF AROCLOR 1260 (8)

RRT[a]	Mean Weight Percent	Relative Std. Dev.[b]	Number of Chlorines[c]	
70	2.7	6.3	5	
84	4.7	1.6	5	
98	3.8	3.5	[d]	
104			5	60%
			6	40%
117	3.3	6.7	6	
125	12.3	3.3	5	15%
			6	85%
146	14.1	3.6	6	
160	4.9	2.2	6	50%
			7	50%
174	12.4	2.7	6	
203	9.3	4.0	6	10%
			7	90%
232	9.8	3.4	[e]	
244			6	10%
			7	90%
280	11.0	2.4	7	
332	4.2	5.0	7	
372	4.0	8.6	8	
448	.6	25.3	8	
528	1.5	10.2	8	
Total	98.6			

[a] Retention time relative to p,p′-DDE = 100. Measured from first appearance of solvent. Overlapping peaks that are quantitated as one peak are bracketed.

[b] Relative standard deviation of six results.

[c] From GC-MS data. Peaks containing mixtures of isomers of different chlorine numbers are bracketed.

[d] Composition determined at the center of peak 104.

[e] Composition determined at the center of peak 232.

inated Hydrocarbons'', *Journal of Chromatography, 70,* 168 (1972).

4. ''Handbook for Analytical Quality Control in Water and Wastewater Laboratories'', Chapter 6, Section 6.4, U. S. Environmental Protection Agency, National Environmental Research Center, Analytical Quality Control Laboratory, Cincinnati, Ohio, 45268, 1972.

5. ''Pesticide Analytical Manual'', U. S. Dept. of Health, Education and Welfare, Food and Drug Administration, Washington, D. C.

6. Bellar, T. A. and Lichtenberg, J. J., ''Method for the Determination of Polychlorinated Biphenyls in Water and Sediment'', U. S. Environmental Protection Agency, National Environmental Research Center, Analytical Quality Control Laboratory, Cincinnati, Ohio, 45268, 1973.

7. Goerlitz, D. F. and Law, L. M., ''Note on Removal of Sulfur Interferences from Sediment Extracts for Pesticide Analysis'', *Bulletin of Environmental Contamination and Toxicology, 6,* 9 (1971).

8. Webb, R. G. and McCall, A. C., ''Quantitative PCB Standards for Electron Capture Gas Chromatography'', *Journal of Chromatographic Science, 11,* 366 (1973).

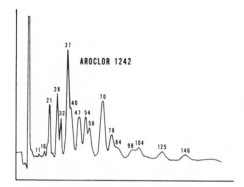

Figure 3. Column: 3% OV-1, Carrier Gas: Nitrogen at 60 ml/min, Column Temperature: 170 C, Detector: Electron Capture.

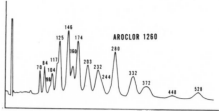

Figure 5. Column: 3% OV-1, Carrier Gas: Nitrogen at 60 ml/min, Column Temperature: 170 C, Detector: Electron Capture.

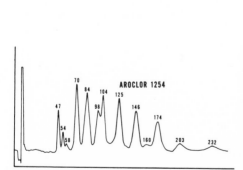

Figure 4. Column: 3% OV-1, Carrier Gas: Nitrogen at 60 ml/min, Column Temperature: 170 C, Detector: Electron Capture.

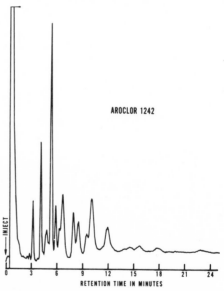

Figure 6. Column: 1.5% OV-17 + 1.95% QF-1, Carrier Gas: Nitrogen at 60 ml/min, Column Temperature: 200 C, Detector: Electron Capture.

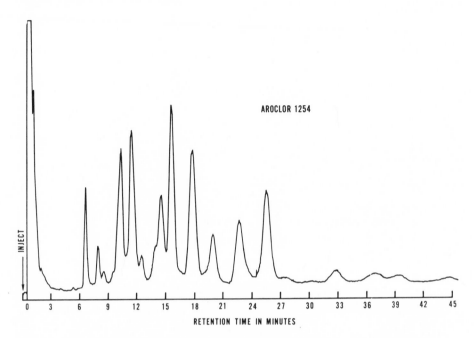

Figure 7. Column : 1.5% OV-17 + 1.95% QF-1, Carrier Gas: Nitrogen at 60 ml/min, Column Temperature: 200 C, Detector: Electron Capture.

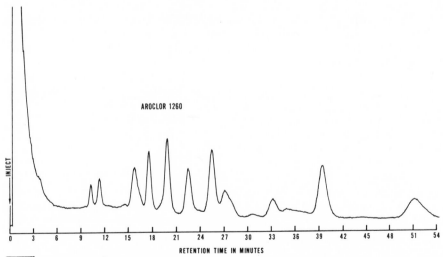

Figure 8. Column: 1.5% OV-17 + 1.95% QF-1, Carrier Gas: Nitrogen at 60 ml/min, Column Temperature: 200C, Detector: Electron Capture

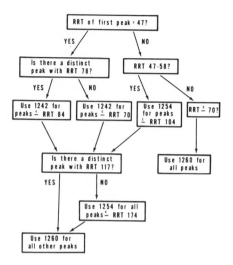

Figure 9. Chromatogram Division Flowchart (8)

Analysis of Trihalomethanes in Drinking Water by Liquid/Liquid Extraction*

1. Scope

1.1 This method (1,2) is applicable only to the determination of four trihalomethanes, i.e., chloroform, bromodichloromethane, chlorodibromomethane, and bromoform in finished drinking water, drinking water during intermediate stages of treatment, and the raw source water.

1.2 For compounds other than the above-mentioned trihalomethanes, or for other sample sources, the analyst must demonstrate the usefulness of the method by collecting precision and accuracy data on actual samples as described in (3) and provide qualitative confirmation of results by Gas Chromatography/Mass Spectrometry (GC/MS) (4).

1.3 Qualitative analyses using GC/MS

or the purge and trap method (5) must be performed to characterize each raw source water if peaks appear as interferences in the raw source analysis.

1.4 The method has been shown to be useful for the trihalomethanes over a concentration range from approximately 0.5 to 200 μg/l. Actual detection limits are highly dependent upon the characteristics of the gas chromatographic system used.

2. Summary

2.1 Ten milliliters of sample are extracted one time with 2 ml of solvent. Three μl of the extract are then injected into a gas chromatograph equipped with a linearized electron capture detector for separation and analysis.

2.2 The extraction and analysis time is 10 to 50 minutes per sample depending

---

* 40 C.F.R. Part 141, Appendix C, Part II.

upon the analytical conditions chosen. (See Table 1 and Figures 1, 2, and 3.)

2.3 Confirmatory evidence is obtained using dissimilar columns and temperature programming. When component concentrations are sufficiently high (>50 μg/l), halogen specific detectors may be employed for improved specificity.

2.4 Unequivocal confirmatory analyses at high levels (>50 μg/l) can be performed using GC/MS in place of the electron capture detector. At levels below 50 μg/l, unequivocal confirmation can only be performed by the purge and trap technique using GC/MS (4, 5).

2.5 Standards dosed into organic free water and the samples are extracted and analyzed in an identical manner in order to compensate for possible extraction losses.

2.6 The concentration of each trihalomethane is summed and reported as total trihalomethanes in μg/l.

3. Interferences

3.1 Impurities contained in the extracting solvent usually account for the majority of the analytical problems. Solvent blanks should be analyzed before a new bottle of solvent is used to extract samples. Indirect daily checks on the extracting solvent are obtained by monitoring the sample blanks (6.4.10). Whenever an interference is noted in the sample blank, the analyst should reanalyze the extracting solvent. The extraction solvent should be discarded whenever a high level (>10 μg/l) of interfering compounds are traced to it. Low level interferences generally can be removed by distillation or column chromatography (6); however, it is generally more economical to obtain a new source of solvent or select one of the approved alternative solvents listed in Section 5.1. Interference-free solvent is defined as a solvent containing less than 0.4 μg/l individual trihalomethane interference. Protect interference-free solvents by storing in a non-laboratory area known to be free of organochlorine solvents. *Subtracting blank values is not recommended.*

3.2 Several instances of accidental sample contamination have been attributed to diffusion of volatile organics through the septum seal on the sample bottle during shipment and storage. The sample blank (6.4.10) is used to monitor for this problem.

3.3 This liquid/liquid extraction technique efficiently extracts a wide boiling range of non-polar organic compounds and, in addition, extracts the polar organic components of the sample with varying efficiencies. In order to perform the trihalomethane analysis as rapdily as possible with sensitivities in the low μg/l range, it is necessary to use the semi-specific electron capture detector and

TABLE 1. RETENTION TIMES FOR TRIHALOMETHANES

Trihalomethane	Retention time minutes		
	Column A	Column B	Column C
Chloroform	1.0	1.3	4.9
Bromodichloromethane	1.5	2.5‖	11.0
Chlorodibromomethane	2.6	5.6	23.1
(Dibromochloromethane) bromoform	5.5	10.9	39.4

‖On this column, trichloroethylene, a common raw source water contaminate, coelutes with bromodichloromethane.

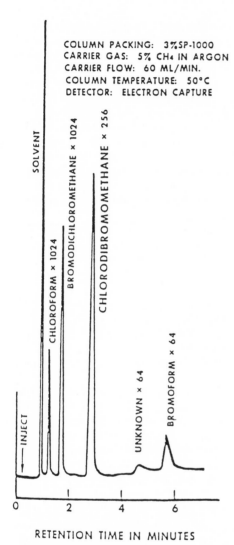

RETENTION TIME IN MINUTES

Figure 1. Finished Water Extract

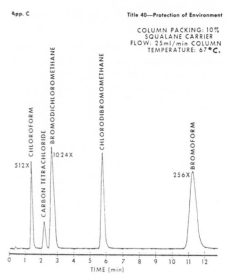

Figure 2. Extract of Standard

chromatographic columns which have relatively poor resolving power. Because of these concessions, the probability of experiencing chromatographic interferences is high. Trihalomethanes are primarily products of the chlorination process and generally do not appear in the raw source water. The absence of peaks in the raw source water analysis with retention times similar to the trihalomethanes is generally adequate evidence of an interference-free finished drinking water analysis. Because of these possible interferences, in addition to each finished drinking water analysis, a representative raw source water (6.4.5) must be analyzed. When potential interferences are noted in the raw source water analysis, the alternate chromatographic columns must be used to reanalyze the sample set. If interferences are still noted, qualitative identifications should be performed according to Sections 2.3 and 2.4. If the peaks are confirmed to be other than trihalomethanes and add significantly to the total trihalomethane value in the finished drinking water analysis, then the sample set must be analyzed by the purge and trap method (5).

4. Apparatus

4.1 Extraction vessel—A 15 ml total volume glass vessel with a Teflon lined screwcap is required to efficiently extract the samples.

4.1.1 For samples that do not form emulsions 10 ml screw-cap flasks with a Teflon faced septum (total volume is ml) are recommended. Flasks and caps— Pierce— #13310 or equivalent. Septa— Teflon silicone—Pierce #12718 or equivalent.

4.1.2 For samples that form emulsions (turbid source water) 15 ml screw cap centrifuge tubes with a Teflon cap liner are recommended. Centrifuge tube—Corning 8062-15 or equivalent.

4.2 Sampling containers—40 ml screw cap sealed with Teflon faced silicone septa. Vials and caps—Pierce #13075 or equivalent. Septa—Pierce #12722 or equivalent.

4.3 Micro syringes—10, 100 μl.

4.4 Micro syringe—25 μl with a 2-inch by 0.006-inch needle—Hamilton 702N or equivalent.

4.5 Syringes—10 ml glass hypodermic with luerlok top (2 each).

4.6 Syringe valve—2-way with luer ends (2 each)—Hamilton #86570—1FM1 or equivalent.

4.7 Pipette—2.0 ml transfer.

4.8 Glass stoppered volumetric flasks— 10 and 100 ml.

4.9 Gas chromatograph with linearized electron capture detector. (Recommended option—temperature programmable. See Section 4.12.)

4.10 Column A—4 mm ID × 2m long glass packed with 3% SP-1000 on Supelcoport (100/120 mesh) operated at 50° C with 60 ml/min flow. (See Figure 1 for a sample chromatogram and Table 1 for retention data.)

4.11 Column B—2 mm ID × 2m long glass packed with 10% squalane on Chromosorb WAW (80/100 mesh) operated at 67° C with 25 ml/min flow. This column is recommended as the primary analytical column. Trichloroethylene, a common raw source water contaminate, coelutes with bromodichloromethane. (See Figure 2 for a sample chromatogram and Table 1 for retention data.)

4.12 Column C—2 mm ID × 3m long glass packed with 6% OV-11/4% SP-2100 on Supelcoport (100/120 mesh) temperature program 45° C for 12 minutes, then program at 1°/minute to 70° C with a 25 ml/min flow. (See Figure 3 for a sample chromatogram and Table 1 for retention data.)

4.13 Standard storage containers—15 ml amber screw-cap septum bottles with Teflon faced silicone septa. Bottles and caps—Pierce #19830 or equivalent. Septa—Pierce #12716 or equivalent.

5. Reagents

5.1 Extraction solvent—(See 3.1). Recommended—Pentane†. Alternative—hexane, methylcyclohexane or 2,2,4-trimethylpentane.

5.2 Methyl alcohol—ACS Reagent Grade.

5.3 Free and combined chlorine reducing agents—Sodium thiosulfate ACS Reagent Grade—sodium sulfite ACS Reagent Grade.

5.4 Activated carbon—Filtrasorb—200, available from Calgon Corporation, Pittsburgh, PA, or equivalent.

5.5 Standards.‡

---

† Pentane has been selected as the best solvent for this analysis because it elutes, on all of the columns, well before any of the trihalomethanes. High altitudes or laboratory temperatures in excess of 75° F may make the use of this solvent impractical. For these reasons, alternative solvents are acceptable; however, the analyst may experience baseline variances in the elution areas of the trihalomethanes due to coelution of these solvents. The degree of difficulty appears to be dependent upon the design and condition of the electron capture detector. Such problems should be insignificant when concentrations of the coeluting trihalomethane are in excess of 5 μg/l.

‡ As a precautionary measure, all standards must be checked for purity by boiling point determinations or GC/MS assays.

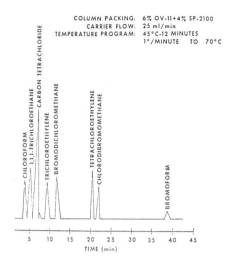

COLUMN PACKING: 6% OV-11+4% SP-2100
CARRIER FLOW: 25 ml/min
TEMPERATURE PROGRAM: 45°C-12 MINUTES
1°/MINUTE TO 70°C

Figure 3. Extract of Standard

5.5.1 Bromoform 96%—available from Aldrich Chemical Company.

5.5.2 Bromodichloromethane 97%—available from Aldrich Chemical Company.

5.5.3 Chlorodibromomethane—available from Columbia Organic Chemicals Company, Inc., 912 Drake Street, Box 9096 E, Columbia, SC, 29208 or Aldrich Chemical Company.

5.5.4 Chloroform 99%—available from Aldrich Chemical Company.

5.6 Organic-free water—Organic-free water is defined as water free of interference when employed in the procedure described herein.

5.6.1 Organic-free water is generated by passing tap water through a carbon filter bed containing carbon. Change the activated carbon whenever the concentration of any trihalomethane exceeds 0.4 $\mu g/l$.

5.6.2 A Millipore Super-Q Water System or its equivalent may be used to generate organic-free deionized water.

5.6.3 Organic-free water may also be prepared by boiling water for 15 minutes.

Subsequently, while maintaining the temperature at 90° C, bubble a contaminant free inert gas through the water at 100 ml/minute for one hour. While still hot, transfer the water to a narrow mouth screw cap bottle with a Teflon seal.

5.6.4 Test organic free water each day it is used by analyzing it according to Section 7.

5.7 Standard stock solutions.

5.7.1 Fill a 10.0 ml ground glass stoppered volumetric flask with approximately 9.8 ml of methyl alcohol.

5.7.2 Allow the flask to stand unstoppered about 10 minutes or until all alcohol wetted surfaces dry.

5.7.3 Weigh the unstoppered flask to the nearest 0.1 mg.

5.7.4 Using a 100 μl syringe, immediately add 2 to 3 drops of the reference standard to the flask, then reweigh. *Be sure that the reference standard falls directly into the alcohol without contacting the neck of the flask.*

5.7.5 Dilute to volume, stopper, then mix by inverting the flask several times.

5.7.6 Transfer the standard solution to a dated and labeled 15 ml screw-cap bottle with a Teflon cap liner.

NOTE.—Because of the toxicity of trihalomethanes, it is necessary to prepare primary dilutions in a hood. It is further recommended that a NIOSH/MESA-approved toxic gas respirator be used when the analyst handles high concentrations of such materials.

5.7.7 Calculate the concentration in micrograms per microliter from the net gain in weight.

5.7.8 Store the solution at 4° C.

NOTE.—All standard solutions prepared in methyl alcohol are stable up to 4 weeks when stored under these conditions. They should be discarded after that time has elapsed.

5.8 Aqueous calibration standard precautions.

5.8.1 In order to prepare accurate aqueous standard solutions, the following precautions must be observed:

a. Do not inject more than 20 μl of alcoholic standards into 100 ml of organic-free water.

b. Use a 25 μl Hamilton 702N microsyringe or equivalent. (Variations in needle geometry will adversely affect the ability to deliver reproducible volumes of methanolic standards into water.)

c. Rapidly inject the alcoholic standard into the expanded area of the filled volumetric flask. Remove the needle as fast as possible after injection.

d. Mix aqueous standards by inverting the flask three times only.

e. Discard the contents contained in the neck of the flask. Fill the sample syringe from the standard solution contained in the expanded area of the flask as directed in Section 7.

f. Never use pipets to dilute or transfer samples and aqueous standards.

g. Aqueous standards, when stored with a headspace, are not stable and should be discarded after one hour. Aqueous standards can be stored according to Sections 6.4.9 and 7.2.

5.9 Calibration standards.

5.9.1 Prepare, from the standard stock solutions a multicomponent secondary dilution mixture in methyl alcohol so that a 20 μl injection into 100 ml of organic-free water will generate a calibration standard which produces a response close ($\pm$ 25%) to that of the unknown. (See 8.1.)

5.9.2 Alternative calibration procedure.

5.9.2.1 Construct a calibration curve for each trihalomethane containing a minimum of 3 different concentrations. Two of the concentrations must bracket each unknown.

5.9.3 Extract and analyze the aqueous calibration standards in the same manner as the unknowns.

5.9.4 Other calibration procedures (7)

which require the delivery of less than 20 μl of methanolic standards to 10.0 ml volumes of water contained in the sample syringe are acceptable only if the methanolic standard is delivered by the solvent flush technique (8).

5.10 Quality Check Standard Mixture.

5.10.1 Prepare, from the standard stock solutions, a secondary dilution mixture in methyl alcohol that contains 10.0 ng/μl of each compound. (See 5.7.6 and 5.7.8.)

5.10.2 Daily, prepare and analyze a 2.0 $\mu g/l$ aqueous dilution from this mixture by dosing 20.0 μl into 100 ml of organic-free water (See Section 8.1).

6. Sample Collection and Handling

6.1 The sample containers should have a total volume of at least 25 ml.

6.1.1 Narrow-mouth screw-cap bottles with the TFE fluorocarbon faced silicone septa cap liners are strongly recommended.

6.2 Glassware Preparation.

6.2.1 Wash all sample bottles, TFE seals, and extraction flasks in detergent. Rinse with tap water and finally with distilled water.

6.2.2 Allow the bottles and seals to air dry, then place in an 105° C oven for 1 hour, then allow to cool in an area known to be free of organics.

NOTE.—Do not heat the TFE seals for extended periods of time (>1 hour) because the silicone layer slowly degrades at 105° C.

6.2.3 When cool, seal the bottles using the TFE seals that will be used for sealing the samples.

6.3 Sample stabilization—A chemical reducing agent (Section 5.3) is added to all samples in order to arrest the formation of additional trihalomethanes after sample collection (7,9) and to eliminate the possibility of free chlorine reacting with impurities in the extraction solvent to form interfering organohalides. *DO NOT ADD*

THE REDUCING AGENT TO SAMPLES AT COLLECTION TIME WHEN DATA FOR MAXIMUM TRIHALOMETHANE FORMATION IS DESIRED. If chemical stabilization is employed, then the reagent is also added to the blanks. The chemical agent (2.5 to 3 mg/40 ml) is added in crystalline form to the empty sample bottle just prior to shipping to the sampling site. If chemical stabilization is not employed at sampling time then the reducing agent is added just before extraction.

6.4 Sample Collection.

6.4.1 Collect all samples in duplicate.

6.4.2 Fill the sample bottles in such a manner that no air bubbles pass through the sample as the bottle is filled.

6.4.3 Seal the bottle so that no air bubbles are entrapped in it.

6.4.4 Maintain the hermetic seal on the sample bottle until analysis.

6.4.5 The raw source water sample history should resemble the finished drinking water. The average retention time of the finished drinking water within the water plant should be taken into account when sampling the raw source water.

6.4.6 Sampling from a water tap.

6.4.6.1 Turn on the water and allow the system to flush until the temperature of the water has stabilized. Adjust the flow to about 500 ml/minute and collect duplicate samples from the flowing stream.

6.4.7 Sampling from an open body of water.

6.4.7.1 Fill a 1-quart wide-mouth bottle with sample from a representative area. Carefully fill duplicate sample bottles from the 1-quart bottle as in 6.4.

6.4.8 If a chemical reducing agent has been added to the sample bottles, fill with sample just to overflowing, seal the bottle, and shake vigorously for 1 minute.

6.4.9 Sealing practice for septum seal screw cap bottles.

6.4.9.1 Open the bottle and fill to overflowing. Place on a level surface. Position

the TFE side of the septum seal upon the convex sample meniscus and seal the bottle by screwing the cap on tightly.

6.4.9.2 Invert the sample and lightly tap the cap on a solid surface. The absence of entrapped air indicates a successful seal. If bubbles are present, open the bottle, add a few additional drops of sample, then reseal bottle as above.

6.4.10 Sample blanks.

6.4.10.1 Prepare blanks in duplicate at the laboratory by filling and sealing sample bottles with organic-free water just prior to shipping the sample bottles to the sampling site.

6.4.10.2 If the sample is to be stabilized, add an identical amount of reducing agent to the blanks.

6.4.10.3 Ship the blanks to and from the sampling site along with the sample bottles.

6.4.10.4 Store the blanks and the samples, collected at a given site (sample set), together in a protected area known to be free from contamination. A sample set is defined as all the samples collected at a given site (i.e., at a water treatment plant, duplicate raw source water, duplicate finished water and the duplicate sample blanks comprise the sample set).

6.5 When samples are collected and stored under these conditions, no measureable loss of trihalomethanes has been detected over extended periods of time (7). It is recommended that the samples be analyzed within 14 days of collection.

7. Extraction and Analysis

7.1 Remove the plungers from two 10-ml syringes and attach a closed syringe valve to each.

7.2 Open the sample bottle[§] (or stan-

[§] If for any reason the chemical reducing agent has not been added to the sample, then it must be added just prior to analyses at the rate of 2.5 to 3 mg/40 ml or by adding 1 mg directly to the sample in the extraction flask.

dard) and carefully pour the sample into one of the syringe barrels until it overflows. Replace the plunger and compress the sample. Open the syringe valve and vent any residue air while adjusting the sample volume to 10.0 ml. Close the valve.

7.3 Fill the second syringe in an identical manner from the same sample bottle. This syringe is reserved for a replicate analysis (see 8.3 and 8.4).

7.4 Pipette 2.0 ml of extraction solvent into a clean extraction flask.

7.5 Carefully inject the contents of the syringe into the extraction flask.

7.6 Seal with a Teflon faced septum.

7.7 Shake vigorously for 1 minute.

7.8 Let stand until the phases separate ($\sim$ 60 seconds).

7.8.1 If the phases do not separate on standing then centrifugation can be used to facilitate separation.

7.9 Analyze the sample by injecting 3.0 μl (solvent flush technique, (8)) of the upper (organic) phase into the gas chromatograph.

8. Analytical Quality Control

8.1 A 2 μg/l quality check standard (See 5.10) should be extracted and analyzed each day before any samples are analyzed. Instrument status checks and lower limit of detection estimations based upon response factor calculations at 5 times the noise level are obtained from these data. In addition, the data obtained from the quality check standard can be used to estimate the concentration of the unknowns. From this information the appropriate standards can be determined.

8.2 Analyze the sample blank and the raw source water to monitor for potential interferences as described in Section 3.1, 3.2, and 3.3.

8.3 Spiked samples.

8.3.1 For those laboratories analyzing more than 10 samples a day, each 10th

sample analyzed should be a laboratory-generated spike which closely duplicates the average finished drinking water in trihalomethane composition and concentration. Prepare the spiked sample in organic-free water as described in section 5.9.

8.3.2 In those laboratories analyzing less than 10 samples daily, each time the analysis is performed, analyze at least one laboratory generated spike sample which closely duplicates the average finished drinking water in trihalomethane composition and concentration. Prepare the spiked sample in organic-free water as described in section 5.9.

8.3.3 Maintain an up-to-date log on the accuracy and precision data collected in Sections 8.3 and 8.4. If results are significantly different than those cited in Section 10.1, the analyst should check out the entire analysis scheme to determine why the laboratory's precision and accuracy limits are greater.

8.4 Randomly select and analyze 10% of all samples in duplicate.

8.5 Analyze all samples in duplicate which appear to deviate more than 30% from any established norm.

8.6 Quarterly, spike an EMSL-Cincinnati trihalomethane quality control sample into organic-free water and analyze.

8.6.1 The results of the EMSL trihalomethane quality control sample should agree within 20% of the true value for each trihalomethane. If they do not, the analyst must check each step in the standard generation procedure to solve the problem.

8.7 It is important that the analyst be aware of the linear response characteristics of the electron capture system that is utilized. Calibration curves should be generated and rechecked quarterly for each trihalomethane over the concentration range encountered in the samples in order to confirm the linear response range of the system. Quantitative data cannot be calculated from non-linear responses.

Whenever non-linear responses are noted, the analyst must dilute the sample for reanalysis.

8.8 Maintain a record of the retention times for each trihalomethane using data gathered from spiked samples and standards.

8.8.1 Daily calculate the average retention time for each trihalomethane and the variance encountered for the analyses.

8.8.2 If individual trihalomethane retention time varies by more than 10% over an eight hour period or does not fall within 10% of an established norm, the system is "out of control." The source of retention data variation must be corrected before acceptable data can be generated.

9. Calculations

9.1 Locate each trihalomethane in the sample chromatogram by comparing the retention time of the suspect peak to the data gathered in 8.8.1. The retention time of the suspect peak must fall within the limits established in 8.8.1 for a single column identification.

9.2 Calculate the concentration of each trihalomethane by comparing the peak heights or peak areas of the samples to those of the standards. Round off the data to two significant figures.

Concentration, $\mu g/l$ = sample peak height/standard peak height $\times$ standard concentration, $\mu g/l$.

9.3 Calculate the total trihalomethane concentration (TTHM) by summing the 4 individual trihalomethane concentrations in $\mu g/l$: TTHM ($\mu g/l$) = (conc. $CHCl_3$) + (conc. $CHBrCl_2$) + (conc. $CHBr_2Cl$) + (conc. $CHBr_3$).

9.4 Calculate the limit of detection (LOD) for each trihalomethane not detected using the following criteria:

$$\text{LOD } (\mu g/l) = \frac{(A \times ATT)}{(B \times ATT) \times (2 \ \mu g/l)}$$

Where:

B = peak height (mm) of 2 $\mu g/l$ quality check standard

A = 5 times the noise level in mm at the exact retention time of the trihalomethane or the base line displacement in mm from theoretical zero at

TABLE 2. SINGLE LABORATORY ACCURACY AND PRECISION

	Dose level $\mu g/l$	Number of samples	Mean $\mu g/l$	Precision relative standard deviation, percent	Accuracy percent recovery
Compound:					
$CHCl_3$	9.1	5	10	11	110
$CHCl_3$	69	3	73	5.3	106
$CHBrCl_2$	1.2	5	1.3	9.8	108
$CHBrCl_2$	12	2	15	1.4	125
$CHBr_2Cl$	2.7	5	2.0	17	74
$CHBr_2Cl$	17	3	16	9.9	94
$CHBr_3$	2.9	5	2.2	10	76
$CHBr_3$	14	3	16	12	114

the exact retention time for the trihalomethane.

ATT = attenuation factor.

9.5 Report the results obtained from the lower limit of detection estimates along with the data for the samples.

10. Precision and Accuracy

10.1 Single lab precision and accuracy. The data in Table 2 were generated by spiking organic-free water with trihalomethanes as described in 5.9. The mixtures were analyzed by the analyst as true unknowns.

References

1. MIEURE, J.P., "A Rapid and Sensitive Method for Determining Volatile Organohalides in Water," *Journal AWWA, 69,* 60, 1977.
2. REDING, R., et al. "THM's in Drinking Water: Analysis by LLE and Comparison to Purge and Trap", Organics Analysis in Water and Wastewater, STP 686 ASTM, 1979.
3. "Handbook for Analytical Quality Control in Water and Waste Water Laboratories,"Analytical Quality Control Laboratory, National Environmental Research Center, Cincinnati, Ohio, June 1972.
4. BUDDE, W.L., J.W. EICHELBERGER, "Organic Analysis Using Gas Chromatography-Mass Spectrometry," Ann Arbor Science, Ann Arbor, Michigan, 1979.
5. "The Analysis of Trihalomethanes in Finished Water by the Purge and Trap Method," Environmental Monitoring and Support Laboratory, Environmental Research Center, Cincinnati, Ohio, 45268, May 15, 1979.
6. RICHARD J.J.; G.A. JUNK, "Liquid Extraction for Rapid Determination of Halomethanes in Water, *Journal AWWA, 69,* 62, January 1977.
7. BRASS, H.J., et al., "National Organic Monitoring Survey: Sampling and Purgeable Organic Compounds, Drinking Water Quality Through Source Protection," R.B. Pojasek, Editor, Ann Arbor Science, p. 398, 1977.
8. WHITE, L.D., et al. "Convenient Optimized Method for the Analysis of Selected Solvent Vapors in Industrial Atmosphere," AIHA Journal, Vol. 31, p. 225, 1970.
9. KOPFLER, F.C., et al. "GC/MS Determination of Volatiles for the National Organics Reconnaissance Survey (NORS) or Drinking Water, Identification and Analysis of Organic Pollutants in Water," L.H. Keith, Editor, Ann Arbor Science, p. 87, 1976.

Determination of Maximum Total Trihalomethane Potential (MTP)*

The water sample used for this determination is taken from a point in the distribution system that reflects maximum residence time. Procedures for sample collection and handling are given in EMSL Methods 501.1 and 501.2. No reducing agent is added to "quench" the chemical reaction producing THMs at the time of sample collection. The intent is to permit the level of THM precursors to be depleted and the concentration of the THMs to be maximized for the supply being tested.

Four experimental parameters affecting maximum THM production are pH, temperature, reaction time and the presence of a disinfectant residual. These parameters are dealt with as follows:

Measure the disinfectant residual at the selected sampling point. Proceed only if a measurable disinfectant residual is present. Collect triplicate 40 ml water samples at the pH prevailing at the time of sam-

---

*40 C.F.R. Part 141, Appendix C, Part III.

pling, and prepare a method blank according to the EMSL methods. Seal and store these samples together for 7 days at 25° C or above. After this time period, open one of the sample containers and check for disinfectant residual. Absence of a disinfectant residual invalidates the sample for further analyses. Once a disinfectant residual has been demonstrated, open another of the sealed samples and determine total THM concentration using either of the EMSL analytical methods.

Method for Volatile Chlorinated Organic Compounds in Water and Wastewaters*

NOTE. — Most of the compounds listed in Para. 1.2 of the following method are determined by Method 514, 15th Edition of *Standard Methods for the Examination of Water and Wastewater,* but the method may be useful for the benezene derivatives.

1. Scope and Application

1.1 This method covers the determination of various chlorinated organic compounds in water and wastewater.

1.2 The following chlorinated organic compounds may be determined individually by this method:
Benzylchloride
Carbon tetrachloride
Chlorobenzene
Chloroform
Epichlorohydrin
Methylene chloride
1,1,2,2-Tetrachloroethane
Tetrachloroethylene
1,2,4-Trichlorobenzene
1,1,2-Trichloroethane

2. Summary

2.1 If the sample is turbid, it is initially centrifuged or filtered through a fiber glass filter in order to remove suspended matter.

A three to ten microliter aliquot of the sample is injected into the gas chromatograph equipped with a halogen specific detector. The resulting chromatogram is used to identify and quantitate specific components in the sample. Results are reported in micrograms per liter. Confirmation of qualitative identifications are made using two or more dissimilar columns.

3. Interferences

3.1 The use of a halogen specific detector minimizes the possibility of interference from compounds not containing chlorine, bromine, or iodine. Compounds containing bromine or iodine will interfere with the determination of organochlorine compounds. The use of two dissimilar chromatographic columns helps to eliminate this interference and, in addition, this procedure helps to verify all qualitative identifications. When concentrations are sufficiently high, unequivocal identifications can be made using infrared or mass spectroscopy. Though non-specific, the flame ionization detector may be used for known systems where interferences are not a problem.

3.2 Ghosting is usually attributed to the history of the chromatographic system.

---

* "Methods for Benzidine, Chlorinated Organic Compounds, Pentachlorophenol and Pesticides in Water and Wastewater" (INTERIM, Pending Issuance of Methods for Organic Analysis of Water and Wastes, September 1978), Environmental Protection Agency, Environmental Monitoring and Support Laboratory (EMSL).

Each time a sample is injected, small amounts of various compounds are adsorbed on active sites in the inlet and at the head of the column. Subsequent injections of water tend to steam clean these sites resulting in non-representative peaks or displacement of the baseline. This phenomenon normally occurs when an analysis of a series of highly concentrated samples is followed by a low level analysis. The system should be checked for ghost peaks prior to each quantitative analysis by injecting distilled water in a manner identical to the sample analysis (1). If excessive ghosting occurs, the following corrective measures should be applied, as required in the order listed:

1) Multiple flushes with distilled water
2) Clean or replace the glass injector liner
3) Replace the chromatographic column

4. Apparatus and Materials

4.1 Gas Chromatograph—Equipped with programmed oven temperature controls and glass-lined injection port. The oven should be equipped with a column exit port and heated transfer line for convenient attachment to the halogen specific detector.

4.2 Detector Options:

4.2.1 Microcoulometric Titration

4.2.2 Electrolytic Conductivity

4.2.3 Flame Ionization

4.3 Recorder—Potentiometric strip chart recorder (10 in) compatible with the detector.

4.4 Syringes—1 μg, 10 μg, and 50 μg.

4.5 BOD type bottle or 40 ml screw cap vials sealed with Teflon faced silicone septa.

4.6 Volumetric Flasks—500 ml, 1000 ml.

4.7 Syringe—Hypodermic Lur-lock type (30 ml).

4.8 Filter glass fiber filter—Type A (13 mm).

4.9 Filter holder—Swinny-type hypodermic adapter (13 mm).

4.10 Glass stoppered ampuls—10 ml.

4.11 Chromatographic columns

4.11.1 Moderately-Polar Column—23 ft × 0.1 in ID × 0.125 in OD stainless steel column #304 packed with 5% Carbowax 20 M on Chromosorb-W (60–80 mesh).

4.11.2 Highly-Polar Column—23 ft × 0.1 in ID × 0.125 in OD stainless steel #304 packed with 5% 1,2,3-Tris-(2-cyanoethoxy) propane on Chromosorb-W (60–80 mesh).

4.11.3 Porous Polymer Column—6 ft × 0.1 in ID × 0.125 in OD stainless steel #304 packed with Chromosorb-101 (60–80 mesh).

4.11.4 Carbopack Column—8 ft × 0.1 in ID × 0.125 in OD stainless steel #304 packed with Carbopack-C (80–100 mesh) + 0.2% Carbowax 1500.

5. Reagents

5.1 Chlorinated hydrocarbon reference standards

5.1.1 Prepare standard mixtures in volumetric flasks using contaminant-free distilled water as solvent. Add a known amount of the chlorinated compounds with a microliter syringe. Calculate the concentration of each component as follows:

$$mg/l = (\text{Density of Compound})(\mu l \text{ injected})$$
$$\times \frac{(1000)}{(\text{Dilution Volume (ml)})}$$

6. Quality Control

6.1 Duplicate quantitative analysis on dissimilar columns should be performed. The duplicate quantitative data should agree within experimental error (±6 percent). If not, analysis on a third dissimilar column should be performed. Spiked sample analyses should be routinely performed to insure the integrity of the method.

7. Selection of Gas Chromatographic Column

7.1 No single column can efficiently resolve all chlorinated hydrocarbons. Therefore, a specific column must be selected to perform a given analysis. Columns providing only partially or non-resolved peaks are useful only for confirmatory identifications. If the qualitative nature of the sample is known, an efficient column selection can be made by reviewing the literature (2). In doing this, one must remember that injection of large volumes of water can cause two serious problems not normally noted using common gas chromatographic techniques:

1) Water can cause early column failure due to liquid phase displacement.

2) Water passing through the column causes retention times and orders to change when compared to common sample solvent media, i.e., hexane or air.

For these reasons, column life and the separations obtained by direct aqueous injection may not be identical to those suggested in literature.

8. Sample Collection and Handling

8.1 The sample containers should have a total volume in excess of 25 to 40 ml, although larger narrow-mouth bottles may be used.

8.1.1 Narrow mouth screw cap bottles with the TFE fluorocarbon face silicone septa cap liners are strongly recommended. Crimp-seal serum vials with TFE fluorocarbon faced septa or ground glass stoppered bottles are acceptable if the seal is properly made and maintained during shipment.

8.2 Sample Bottle Preparation

8.2.1 Wash all sample bottles and TFE seals in detergent. Rinse with tap water and finally with distilled water.

8.2.2 Allow the bottles and seals to air dry at room temperature.

8.2.3 Place the bottle in a 200° C oven for one hour, then allow to cool in an area known to be free of organics.

8.2.4 When cool, seal the bottles using the TFE seals that will be used for sealing the samples.

8.3 The sample is best preserved by protecting it from phase separation. Since the majority of the chlorinated solvents are volatile and relatively insoluble in water, it is important that the sample bottle be filled completely to minimize air space over the sample. Acidification will minimize the formation of nonvolatile salts formed from chloroorganic acids and certain chlorophenols. However, it may interfere with the detection of acid degradable compounds such as chloroesters. Therefore, the sample history must be known before any chemical or physical preservation steps can be applied. To insure sample integrity, it is best to analyze the sample within 1 hour of collection.

8.4 Collect all samples in duplicate.

8.5 Fill the sample bottles in such a manner that no air bubbles pass through the sample as the bottle is filled.

8.6 Seal the bottles so that no air bubbles are entrapped in it.

8.7 Maintain the hermetic seal on the sample bottle until analysis.

8.8 Sampling from a water tap.

8.8.1 Turn on water and allow the system to flush. When the temperature of the water has stabilized, adjust the flow to about 500-ml/minute and collect duplicate samples from the flowing stream.

8.9 Sampling from an open body of water.

8.9.1 Fill a 1-quart wide-mouth bottle with sample from a representative area. Carefully fill duplicate 25 to 40 ml-sample bottles from the 1-quart bottle.

9. Sample Preparation

9.1 If the sample is turbid, it should be filtered or centrifuged to prevent syringe plugging or excessive ghosting problems. Filtering the sample is accomplished by filling a 30-ml hypodermic syringe with sample and attaching the Swinny-type hypodermic filter adaptor with a glass fiber filter "Type A" installed. Discard the first 5 ml of sample then collect the filtered sample in a glass stoppered sample bottle filled to the top. (One should occasionally analyze the non-filtered sample to insure that the filtering technique does not adversely affect the sample).

10. Method of Analysis

10.1 Daily, analyze a standard containing 10.0 mg/l of each compound to be analyzed as a quality check sample before any samples are analyzed. Instrument status checks and lower limit of detection estimations based upon response factor calculations at two times the signal to noise ratio are obtained from these data. In addition, response factor data obtained from this standard can be used to estimate the concentration of the unknowns.

10.2 Analyze the filtered sample of unknown composition by injecting 3 to 10 μl into the gas chromatograph. Record the injection volume and detector sensitivity.

10.3 Prepare a standard mixture consisting of the same compounds in concentrations approximately equal to those detected in the sample. Chromatograph the standard mixture under conditions identical to the unknown.

11. Calculation of Results

11.1 Measure the area of each unknown peak and each reference standard peak as follows:

Area = (Peak Height) (Width of Peak at 1/2 Height)

11.2 Calculate the concentration of each unknown as follows:

$$mg/l = \frac{(\text{Area of Sample peak}) (\mu l \text{ of Standard Injected}) (\text{Conc'n of Standard})}{(\mu l \text{ of Sample injected}) (\text{Area of Standard Peak})}$$

12. Reporting Results

12.1 Report results in mg/l. If a result is negative, report the minimum detectable limit (see 10.1). When duplicate and spiked samples are analyzed, all data obtained should be reported.

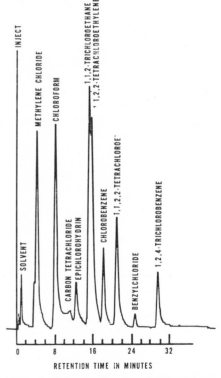

Figure 1. Column: Chromosorb-101, Temperature Program: 125C for 4 min then 4C/min up to 280C., Carrier Gas: Nitrogen at 36 ml/min, Detector: Microcoulometric.

References

1. Dressman, R.C., "Elimination of Memory Peaks Encountered in Aqueous-Injection Gas Chromatography," *Journal of Chromatographic Science, 8,* 265 (1970).

2. "Gas Chromatography Abstracts," Knapman, C.E.H., Editor, Institute of Petroleum, 61 New Cavendish Street, London W1M8AR, Annually 1958 to date, since 1970, also includes Liquid Chromatography Abstracts.